£19.95

D1608598

HOMESICKNESS, COGNITION, AND HEALTH

Homesickness, Cognition, and Health

Shirley Fisher

Centre for Occupational and Health Psychology
Department of Psychology
The University of Strathclyde
Glasgow, Scotland

LAWRENCE ERLBAUM ASSOCIATES, PUBLISHERS
Hove and London (UK)   Hillsdale (USA)

Lawrence Erlbaum Associates Ltd., Publishers
27 Palmeira Mansions
Church Road
Hove
East Sussex, BN3 2FA
U.K.

British Library Cataloguing in Publication Data

Fisher, Shirley
    Homesickness, cognition, and health.
    1. Homesickness.
    I. Title.
    155.9

    ISBN 0-86377-120-3

Typeset by Acorn Bookwork, Salisbury, Wiltshire
Printed and bound by BPCC Wheatons, Exeter

Contents

To Reg Pittman

Acknowledgements

The work reported in this book was supported by funds from the Social Science Research Council and by the Manpower Services Commission.

I would like to thank Alan Wilkes of the Department of Psychology, The University of Dundee for all the helpful comments and discussions during the writing of this book. I would also like to thank Ms Marilyn Laird for typing the manuscript and Ms Rohays Perry of Lawrence Erlbaum Associates for help with the processes of production. Finally, I would like to thank my husband, Reg Pittman, for his tolerance and help during the preparation of the manuscript.

Preface

Homesickness is a topic which has been largely unresearched in spite of the fact that it may be associated with marked distress in some individuals and that research results are likely to be of considerable interest for all those who have counselling or care-giving roles with respect to those who have left home to become newly residential.

Dictionary definitions of homesickness include 'pining for home' *(Chambers Twentieth Century Dictionary)* and 'depressed by absence from home' *(Concise Oxford English Dictionary)*. Dictionary definitions do not, however, provide any indication of the range of symptoms likely to be associated with the experience. Although some 17th century medical texts identified physical ailments associated with the move from home (see Chapter 3), there has been little exploration of the topic and its associated symptoms in modern research.

GENERAL FEATURES OF THE BOOK

This book represents the culmination of a research effort funded by the Economic and Social Science Research Council and by the Manpower Services Commission, involving three years of research in selected schools, universities, and colleges. The main drive of the research was to examine the psychological effects of the transition to an institution for secondary or tertiary education or for vocational training. Of central interest was the nature and incidence of self-reported homesickness.

Although the range of populations involved in leaving home is potentially great it was necessary to be selective in the investigations. Research was therefore confined to populations of boarding school children (residents at establishments offering fee-paying secondary education), university students, and student nurses attending college in teaching hospitals. Investigations of university students were not confined to the University of Dundee, but we thought it prudent not to mention specifically the universities involved. There have now been sufficient studies in different locations for us to conclude that the main findings reported in this volume have generality. As noted earlier, there are many other situations where a person leaves home to reside elsewhere; it was impossible to study the wide range of reasons and circumstances attached to such decisions. In this sense, the body of work reported in this volume is specific.

Although all subjects studied were able to provide written definitions of the term 'homesickness', only about 18–20% spontaneously use the term when asked to list stressful problems in the first term of the first year in an institution. If the term is provided for endorsement, about two-thirds of most populations studied, self-report the experience by endorsing the appropriate cell on a category rating scale. Contrary to popular expectations, we found little evidence of sex or age differences within the populations studied. Of those who report the experience about 10–15% are seriously disturbed and report themselves as continuously homesick when provided with a 12- or 24-hour grid marked against a time scale.

In the process of investigating the occurrence of homesickness, the stresses encountered by all students making the transition to university or nursing college became evident. Manifest forms of distress included depression, obsessionality, somatic symptom reporting, phobic avoidance, and absent-mindedness. Clearly the transition to university is a profound and sometimes quite negative experience for students. It should perhaps be emphasised that this is not true for all students; the intriguing issues concern the definition of the differentiating factors.

In 16th and 17th century medical texts on homesickness, the issue was raised of whether the environment was the important factor or whether there were vulnerable personality traits. This issue is addressed but not answered completely in this book; we have located some very powerful forms of environmental influence but we have also found some evidence to suggest that there may be individuals who are vulnerable in that they differ from their non-homesick counterparts prior to leaving home.

A second issue of particular interest is the predominance of distressing ruminative activity in the thinking and attention of the homesick. At the extreme, the person who is very homesick appears quite overwhelmed by constant preoccupation with thoughts of home. The mildly homesick person appears less continuously preoccupied and such periods are confined to episodes. Nevertheless, the cognitive state of homesickness seems to be characterised by profound and frequent domination of attention by home-related ruminations. It appears that the focus of attentional concern is not problems generated at home or arising because of leaving home, but is more likely to be uncontrollable ideations concerned with home. These issues are of considerable theoretical interest in the understanding of the rules of planning process; could it be that the very nature of planned activity involves strong dominance of plans in memory to such an extent that they can continue to dominate the internal focus of attention long after they have ceased to be appropriate? In the case of bereavement, it might be appropriate to ask whether it is possible not to think constantly of the deceased; in the case of homesickness it might be reasonable to ask under what circumstances a person would be able to direct his or her thoughts away from home.

THE THEORETICAL BASIS OF HOMESICKNESS

A number of theories have been identified that account for some of the components of homesickness. There are two principal elements of interest; the first is the dominance in attentional focus of home-related ruminative activity and the second concerns the symptoms which accompany the experience.

It was clear from the outset that we were not easily going to be able to provide a final test of the competing theories in terms of the form and manifestation of homesickness. There may be many causes of psychological distress and yet a limit to the form that the symptoms can take. Nevertheless there are some differences in the predictions in that some favour anxiety as the predominant initial reaction whereas others favour depression.

Most readers will be familiar with the effects of separation and loss as described by Bowlby (1969; 1973; 1980). The infant when deprived of visual contact with its mother shows signs of anxiety, panic and searching behaviour. The similarity with the anxious searching and panic of the recently bereaved (Parkes, 1972) raises the issue of whether there is a basic biological process which serves to raise anxiety in cases of loss of a loved person. The loss model would suppose the homesick to be temporarily bereaved, suffering acute anxiety and panic because of loss of direct contact with home and family; the predominant distress symptom should be anxiety. Preoccupation with thoughts of home should also be characteristic.

Interruption theory proposed by Mandler (1975) would also predict raised anxiety and preoccupation with thoughts of home but for different reasons. Mandler's theory assumes that interruption of on-going activity creates release of tension because this is part of the impetus contained in planned activity. Therefore, blocked or thwarted behaviour creates irritation and even anxiety if substitute activity cannot be found. Although based on laboratory research, Mandler notes the relevance for understanding the stress created by life events; interruption is often a common denominator. As leaving home inevitably results in the breaking of old familiar routines raised anxiety might be a predicted consequence.

The control theory proposed by Fisher (1986) hypothesise that the transition from a familiar to a new environment results in a period of loss of control. A person who is skilled at dealing with the demands of his or her life prior to transition suddenly becomes helpless in a new location. In the case of joining a new educational establishment, helplessness might be more profound because of the difficulties associated with coping with new academic and social demands as well as with new locations and daily routines. It would be expected that depression might be more characteristic than anxiety following the transition from home. Control theory copes less well with preoccupation with the 'old' or home environment; the emphasis should be on the new environment.

Finally, there is the theory that transition inevitably results in a change in role; a person who moves from home to college assumes the role of college student as compared with the role at home of son or daughter or school pupil. Adapting to the new role results in a period of anxiety in which self-focused attention predominates (Wapner, Kaplan, & Ciottone, 1981; Oatley, 1988). These theories and other related theories are examined in more detail in the early chapters of this book. Most predict that the prime symptom which interacts with the transition for the homesick is anxiety. There is some evidence to support this but also other evidence to support the fact that the experience creates raised depression for all students.

THE IMPORTANCE OF THE POST-TRANSITION ENVIRONMENT

As the research proceeded it became clear that the new or post-transition environment has a fundamental moderating role in controlling the occurrence of self-reported episodes of homesickness. This may be because of the encouragement of personal commitment to a new way of life if the new environment is perceived as attractive. However, it may also be the case that the new environment creates unpleasant experiences such as 'job strain'. Towards the end of the book we review the evidence which suggests that homesickness may be a secondary phenomenon; a response to the perceived strains of the new environment. This perception creates the need for mental 'escapism' which means that thoughts of home are voluntarily selected. The distress penalty that the pleasure of nostalgia brings is in one sense comparable with the unpleasant side-effects of taking a drug.

THE STRUCTURE OF THE BOOK

The book is organised in such a way as to provide first the factual information about homesickness from research studies and then to progress towards theoretical understanding. It is intended that the book will be read not only by academics and researchers who are interested in the causes and consequence of grief-related ruminative activity, but also by counsellors and those in authority or care-giving roles. For this reason we have attempted to provide the information in a form which helps it to be assembled easily.

The first part of the book is concerned with identifying the theoretical bases of the effects of relocations and with identifying some of the theoretical explanations for such effects. In particular, loss models, interruption, control, and role models are considered. The central part of the book is concerned with specifying the incidence, phenomenology, and moderating factors in homesickness. Later there is consideration of the consequences for mental and physical health. The final part of the book is concerned with consideration of conceptual models of homesickness. The main emphasis is on understanding how cognition is so organised that 'nostalgic thoughts' from the pre-transition environment come to dominate cognitive activity, provide intrusion into daily life, and are associated with distress symptoms.

The implications for therapy and intervention are considered towards the end of the book. Cognitive theorists may find these considerations of theoretical interest. It is, however, hoped that the practical orientation will provide some guides for those who are medical practitioners, psychiatrists, and counsellors who need to deal with the distress associated with homesickness.

In the Appendix, a method of measuring and assessing homesickness is provided. The inventory was developed as a result of three years research by Fisher and Murray involving students from four universities. Conventional techniques for validation were difficult because of the difficulty of trying to assess a state rather than a trait and because of the lack of a criterion group independently diagnosed. The inventory is short (26 items) and correlates well with self-assessed homesickness. It is hoped that it may prove useful as a diagnostic device. The indication for its use would be a recent move away from home and physical disorders or psychological disturbance.

1
Geographical Transitions:
Context-Dependent Effects
and the Concept of
Congruence

The purpose of this chapter is to consider some of the background research literature on the effects of relocation and migration on mental and physical health. The chapter provides the background for understanding the importance of relocation in the lives of individuals. On first consideration, the evidence supports an association between relocations and vulnerability to ill health. However, there are a number of methodological difficulties with the interpretation of the evidence. In most cases where a positive association is reported, there is the confounding effect of downward mobility or the difficulty of self-selection factors. Taken collectively, however, there is a strong case for arguing that there is an apparent associative link between mobility and mental health or physical disorder. The relationship needs unpacking with the help of studies focused on specific psychological effects.

THE HISTORY OF RESEARCH INTO GEOGRAPHICAL MOVES

The history of research into the effects of geographical transitions suggests that they are stressful and likely to increase the risk of mental or physical disorder. The scale designed by Holmes and Rahe (1965), which provides an order of magnitude of the stressful qualities of life events, indicates that geographical moves ('major change in residence') are listed 24th on the rank order list of stressful life events as assessed from the ratings of healthy Americans. The finding that clinically depressed patients rate moving as the third of the most important factors in their recent life history, prior to the onset of depression (Leff, Roatch, & Bunney, 1970), might imply that moves feature more prominently as major life events. But it might also be argued that since only clinical populations were involved in the study, the importance of moves might only be high for those already vulnerable in some way.

The above analysis hints at the importance of contexts and personal meanings as determinants of the weighting a person gives to a particular life event. Geographical moves may be of more significance to some individuals because of personal life history or because of personality dispositions. Fisher (1988a) argues that in order to understand the relationship between life events and disorder, it is necessary to take account of mediating variables such as control, self-esteem, and attributional style, as well as mood state at the time the assessment is made. These variables or their absence may constitute vulnerability or fortitude factors respectively. Clearly, what is needed is some attempt to weigh up contextual and personality factors in determining the impact of geographical transitions. Exactly the same argument is true for analysis of the impact of all forms of life events on health and welfare. However, attempts to provide weighting of contexts in assessing the relationship between life events and disorder, although desirable, produce difficulties because of the need for semi-structured interviews which may constrain the reports given by subjects and because of the subjectivity involved when contextual detail is judged (see Brown, 1974).

Migration and Health

The research literature on relocation and migration has, over the years, provided a very strong indication of a relationship with poor mental and physical health. However, there are a number of difficulties with the interpretation of the research findings. Correlations do not imply causation; more car drivers who wear seat-belts are involved in car accidents but this should not be taken to imply that wearing a seat-belt causes a car accident. Equally, even when the causal link can be established, the direction of causation remains unknown; A may cause B, B may cause A, or there may be some third factor which influences both A and B. These considerations are important because although there is a tendency to attribute the causes of ill health to the geographical transition, self-selection factors may be operative (those who move away may be those who are poor or discontented with a previous environment).

A number of early studies focused on the health of migrant communities as compared with that of the indigenous population. For example, Odegaard (1932) reported greater rates of hospital admissions for mental disorder amongst Norwegian immigrants to Minnesota than for either the native-born of Minnesota or Norway. Malzberg and Lee (1940) reported a similar result for populations in New York when age, colour, and sex were taken into account. These studies, although not devoid of the above-stated methodological difficulties, point to the vulnerability of the migrant group. The reasons for the effect remain unclear; there may have been exposure to adverse environments, mediating behaviours may increase the risk of ill health, general poverty factors may weaken resources through poor nutrition, etc.

However there is also evidence against the hypothesis of vulnerability of the migrant with regards to mental disorder. Thus, Kleiner and Parker (1963) demonstrated the greater prevalence of psychoneurotic and psychosomatic symptoms in native-born individuals migrating within the U.S.A. There was some evidence of greater discrepancy between educational aspiration and achievement for the native-born group. There were no differences between the migrant or native-born groups in terms of status inconsistency. These studies also underlined the possible importance of circumstantial factors in that the discrepancy between education and achievement was greater for the native-born migrant groups.

Perhaps the most quoted work which also underlines the confounding of circumstantial factors with the effects of mobility, is that of Faris and Dunham (1939) who, using home ownership as an index of stability and rental status as an index of mobility in the city of Chicago, found a negative association with mobility and mental health. The mobile areas of cities were also, however, most socially disorganised and most likely to be associated with poverty. The conclusion that social location may be the cause of psychopathology epitomises the main difficulties of interpretation. As is now well understood, those with poor mental health may become incompetent and drift down to ghetto areas of cities; equally the stress of these areas may create the nurturent conditions for psychopathology. With regard to the issue of whether or not moving and migration are stressful *per se*, the study merely underlines the close association with poverty, social class, lack of educational and social mobility in such cases. Thus, moves may reflect or create underlying conditions associated with psychopathology. Moves and contexts seem inextricably linked.

The picture is much the same with physical health. Research evidence across the last 60 years has demonstrated the vulnerability of migrant populations to physical ill health. In particular, cardiovascular disease, gastric disorders, and infectious illnesses such as tuberculosis have been found to be more prevalent in migrant populations than in the 'initial' or 'receiving' communities (see Medalie & Kahn, 1973; Cruze-Coke, Etcheverry & Nagel, 1964; Wolff, 1953; Christenson & Hinkle, 1961). In most of these studies the problem of the confounding of the stressful effects of moving with both the circumstances which engender it and the situations which result, remains a problem. Migration may also create intermediate conditions of crowding, poor sanitation, and so on, or may create fatigue and lowered resistance. A further difficulty is that moving may provide a focus for the reporting of existing symptoms.

In general, the migration studies hint at the possibility of the existence of stress-related factors creating poor mental and physical health, but do not provide sufficient detail concerning the immediate responses resulting from migration and moving.

Specific Effects of Relocation

In order to identify the effects of transition on mental and physical health, examination of psychological changes following the move is an advantage. Unfortunately, there have not been many studies of this nature, but one useful study was carried out by Fried (1962) who examined the reaction of slum dwellers to enforced moves into better housing within a city, as part of a slum clearance scheme. If anything, the circumstances surrounding the move should have been perceived as positive. There was the possibility of upward social mobility to better housing in a better district. However, pre- and post-relocation interviews showed that psychological reactions were intense, overwhelming, prolonged, and characterised by grief for home: 'I felt as if the heart was taken out of me' (p. 347). Depressive mood and a sense of helplessness were major features of the observed reaction following the move.

Fried's study also emphasised the central importance of objects and places as critical factors; those who moved to new housing reported missing loved home fixtures and reported returning to look at the house because of all the happy memories. Perhaps objects symbolically represent memories or perhaps they become coveted and loved possessions in their own right because of their familiar presence in the home. The role of situational and personal factors was evident. Status, defined by occupational, educational, and income factors was positively associated with successful adjustment, 72% of the higher-income group adjusted successfully to the move as compared with 22% of their lower-income counterparts.

Planning for the move appears to be a critical factor although it may reflect underlying factors associated with willingness to adjust; 52% who reported planning for the move were subsequently found to have adjusted well, as compared with 24% of those who, if anything, reported resisting the move. Fried developed the idea of 'preparedness for transition' as a critical determinant of the success of adaptation. 'Mastery' defined in terms of the determination to struggle and persist against all envisaged problems was seen as a sign of 'inner preparedness' for the impending move.

More recent studies of relocation tend to have been concerned not with enforced conditions (as in slum clearance) but with the naturally occurring voluntary moves undertaken by individuals during their lives. Two points of view exist. The first is that moving is stressful, unpleasant and has to be coped with because of the necessities of upward mobility. The other is that moving is a positive process resulting in new experiences and encounters. Demographic trends in the U.S.A. indicate that about 20% of the population are mobile and that many people do accomplish moves voluntarily and without becoming ill. Fischer and Stueve (1977) conclude that only those individuals affected by poverty, racial discrimination, or physical infirmity are likely to be vulnerable to adverse effects.

Perhaps contextual and personal factors operate to influence outcome and, thus, both positions could be valid. What may be important is willingness to change cultural and social outlook and to become committed to a new place. Syme (1967) describes the process of going through these changes as 'cultural mobility' and envisages the changes as influencing the disease risk. An interesting outcome of a longitudinal study on the effects of relocation by Stokols, Schumaker, and Martinez (1983) was an indication that even though mobility might be the fashion for a vigorous, modern economic nation, moving may have negative implications. The study involved 242 adult employees, 121 of whom completed a follow-up study of emotional and physical well being three months after a move to a new job in a new location. The authors obtained self-report data on mobility history and reported that frequent relocation was associated with a greater number of illness-related symptoms and reduced satisfaction. The study indicated the adverse effect of moves on those with 'low exploratory tendency'; this was described in terms of lack of exploration of various aspects of the psychosocial environment. This is an interesting finding because, as will be argued later in the book, commitment to new sources of information may be a very important prerequisite of adjustment.

The study also showed that raised illness symptoms were present in those who had low mobility history but who perceived low choice of residence and low congruence with expectations. This suggests that explanation of mobility history and its relationship with success and happiness post relocation is complex. Both low mobility and high mobility groups may be more at risk for adverse experience than moderate mobility groups.

Fisher, Frazer, and Murray (1986), and Fisher and Hood (1988) have produced evidence to show that some aspects of previous mobility experience may protect against adverse reaction to the move away from home in both university students and boarding school populations. In particular, previous experience away from home at an institution reduces the risk of homesickness reporting. Again the issue of interest is whether we are dealing with a self-selection factor (perhaps those who have good experiences on leaving home are more willing to move to a new environment), or whether benefits occur because resources are acquired and a person learns how to deal with a new environment when separated from the security and support from home. These issues will be dealt with in later chapters.

CONTEXTUAL FACTORS AND PERSONAL DECISION

Since human responses in relation to anticipated events may involve planning and exploration in advance (see Fisher 1986, Chapter 7), contextual factors might operate on the decision to move, as well as on decisions as to whether or not the move is perceived as resulting in satisfactory and positive experiences. The irreversible nature of some moves may give the early decision making particular potency and create a period of stress in advance.

At this early stage in decision making, variables such as economic and social advantage may be weighed against the advantages of remaining in the current place. The 'push' and 'pull' of the situation may need to be assessed over a period of time. The individual may thus be information-seeking and might be expected to be preoccupied.

The Cogruence Model of Relocation

Stokols (1979) developed a congruence analysis of human stress in which the important factor is 'environment-behaviour' congruence, or the extent to which a particular environment meets the needs of a particular person. It is defined in terms of two measurable elements; the first is controllability and the second is salience. A further useful distinction made by Stokols is between experiential congruence (or the degree to which the environment objectively meets a person's needs), and mental congruence or how well the environment actually accommodates the characteristics and behaviour of the person (Michelson, 1976).

Stokols notes the importance of hierarchically ordered concerns. For example, physical safety and emotional security are foremost followed by environmental constraints and supports etc. It is assumed that when higher order concerns are not threatened or relevant, lower order concerns become more salient.

With regard to the effects of contexts on the response to moves, the important point is that contextual factors may provide: (a) the basis of the decision to move; and (b) the context in which the impact of the move is evaluated. A person may base the decision to move on anticipated benefits and weight these against the costs. If after the transition these conditions are not what was expected, a situation of incongruence is created. Also the objective and subjectively perceived aspect of the situation may be discrepant; a person may perceive a pleasant environment in negative terms because he or she did not want to move or feels depressed. All these factors are likely to affect commitment.

The congruence model provides some reconciliation of the view that moves have both positive and negative features and that personal factors may selectively highlight various aspects of moving.

Person-environment Fit in Work Environments

In the context of examining stress in working environments, French, Caplan, and Van Harrison (1982) formulated the concept of person-environment congruence. The characteristics of the person and the environment as objectively defined, constitute objective congruence. The subjectively perceived properties of the environment and the objective environment, constitute level of perceived congruence. French et al. reported that perceived congruence is related to mental and physical health in occupational settings in the form of a 'U' relationship.

These issues are returned to later in the book but in the context of the issue of the effects of relocation, these models allow scope for differences in individual reaction as well as providing a basis for understanding environmental influences. Each move may result in beneficial or adverse effects as a function of circumstances, personal preferences, and meanings attributed by individuals.

Figure 1.1, on page 8, illustrates the possible ways in which relocations as life events may link with physical health. First, there may be the creation of adverse environmental conditions. Secondly, there may be behavioural links which increase the risk of encounters with disease agents or which involve abuse of bodily systems. Thirdly, there may be stress effects because of the instability of moving. These stress effects may create a hormone climate in which the immune system is suppressed or in which chronic disease is more likely because of functional abuse of bodily systems.

SUMMARY AND CONCLUSIONS

The investigations of migration and mobility have indicated that there appears to be a strong relationship between relocations and ill health. However there are many confounding variables which make interpretation of the evidence difficult. What is needed are studies which unpack some of the issues by focusing on the psychological effects of major moves in individuals. Models which emphasise the importance of congruence or fit between the person and the environment provide a basis for understanding psychological effects in terms of both environmental context and personal factors in cognition.

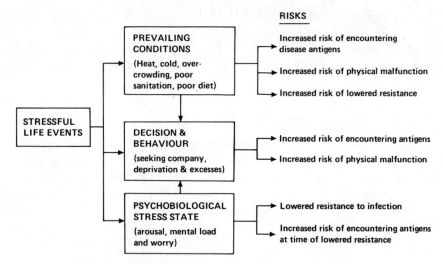

FIG. 1.1.   Conceptual model of factors increasing the risk of disease following a stressful life event—e.g. migration, relocation, bereavement, marital separation, and divorce (Fisher 1988, with kind permission of John Wiley & Sons).

2 Theories of the Psychological Effects of Change and Transition

The previous chapter was concerned with the adverse effects of relocations on health. Although, as illustrated by Fig. 1.1, relocations may create circumstances which favour ill health, one possible explanation for ill health following moves is that they create periods of stress. If relocations are stressful, the interesting issue is why they are stressful and how this might translate into poor health risk.

A common denominator of all types of relocations is that change and transition are involved. Yet change and transition are recurring features of modern life. Man could be argued to have as part of his psychological make-up the adaptive capacity for coping with new environments and new experiences. There are some kinds of life events which are negative and which have a profound adverse effect on human psychological function; these are the events characterised by loss. Of particular significance in this respect are changes which involve loss of a loved person, object or environment. The profound effect of, for example, bereavement has been well documented (Parkes, 1972). Environmental relocations may involve all three of these sorts of losses and although the loss may be temporary and communication remains possible, still the psychological effects associated with loss may be paramount. This is particularly true when relocation is of the form which involves leaving home to reside in a new place. Many young people face relocations of this sort, often because of the opportunity for further education and vocational training.

This book concentrates on leaving home as a particularly stressful form of relocation and the form most frequently associated with homesickness and distress. The book is addressed to the issue of the psychological and physical response to moves away from home and incorporates the results of three years of research in schools, nursing colleges and universities. The distress pattern associated with leaving home to live and work in another environment is commonly termed 'homesickness'. In spite of the fact that a definition of homesickness exists in most dictionaries and languages, and that the term is well understood by those employed in supervisory and administrative capacities in boarding schools and universities, there has been little systematic research on the topic.

EXPLANATIONS OF THE EFFECTS OF TRANSITIONS FROM HOME

Loss and Grief

On first consideration, the most appropriate theoretical format for understanding the effects of leaving home would seem to be that of attachment and loss. The death of a loved person such as a parent or spouse is a significant stressful experience for most of those who experience it. The Social Readjustment Rating Scale (Holmes & Rahe, 1965), introduced to quantify the level of stress associated with life events, was based on the arithmetic weightings provided by normal subjects given an arbitrary value of 50 for 'marriage'. Other events were then rated relative to marriage. Death of a spouse was given a value of 100 and was top of the list of stressful life events. On this scale, relocation was much less stressful than bereavement: change in residence or living conditions was given a score of 20 and change to a new job was given a value of 36. Leaving home was not separately rated and so there is no indication of how stressful normal people would find this.

In terms of the life event scale, relocations are less threatening than events such as bereavement and, therefore, this would imply that the same degree of loss cannot be involved. However this does not mean that some element of loss might not be involved in leaving home. The difference is of course that it will be perceived as reversible as compared with bereavement where loss is irreversible. The ability of human beings to know and represent the continued existence of home may be the critical factor. Nevertheless, the break in contact with home may be expected to create partial bereavement. There may be similar features in the loss experience.

Death may have an impact on the bereaved for a number of reasons. Loss involves the termination of a close relationship but simultaneously involves a change of life-style and may involve a sequence of threatening events such as financial insecurity and loss of friends. For those who write about the phenomenology, it is the total loss of the relationship with another person which is of paramount importance. One issue of interest is whether the response to death of a loved person has a biological basis (medical model) or is a psychological phenomenon. Studies by Bowlby (1969; 1973; 1980) have probed the basis of the reaction to loss of immediate contact between mother and child and indicate that the maintenance of a close bond between child and parents creates a sense of security and is itself sought at time of stress. The infant reacts with alarm characterised by protest, searching, and distress when there is no visual contact with the mother.

Lest it seems inappropriate to extrapolate from findings concerning infants deprived of their mothers to the case of the bereaved adult, Weiss (1975; 1978; 1982) has investigated attachment behaviour in adults and has indicated that relationships between parent and adult offspring, or between close friends, may have similar properties to the mother-infant bond. Caretaker relationships are likely to evolve in most close bonds. Weiss notes the similarity of the response to loss at all ages and sees this as suggesting the operation of a single perceptual-emotional system.

If the response to leaving home could be considered as a reversible bereavement, it is useful to ask what properties we would expect to find in the response pattern which results. Bowlby (1980) itemises four phases of bereavement. First there is a phase of numbing that lasts for a few hours to a week, and may be accompanied by outbursts of panic or anger. There is then a 'yearning phase' characterised by searching for the lost person. This phase can last for years. There is then a phase of disorganisation and despair. This is followed by a final phase of reorganisation.

Parkes (1972) identified four elements of search behaviour. The first is the pining stage in which preoccupation with thoughts of the deceased occurs. The second involves attentional focus on places and objects associated with the lost person. The third involves misinterpreting signs and cues as representing the deceased. The fourth involves calling out or bursting into tears in ways perhaps reminiscent of the distress of the infant.

There are two reasons why it would be inappropriate to expect to find stages in the response to leaving home which model the stages of bereavement. First, although appealing because of the ease with which stages in the response to loss can be indentified, it has been argued that clear and invariant sequences of behaviour are not obvious as part of the grief reaction; people sometimes move backwards through stages. Thus the parallel with developmental sequence is not apparent (see Bugen, 1977). Secondly, leaving home is not a permanent break with home; in fact home may be contacted and is usually frequently visited; the acute sense of total loss should be less likely. Nevertheless, boarding school children do cry on the way to boarding school and anxious 'grief-like' reactions seem typical of the distress at leaving home for some people.

The response to bereavement is profound and may affect physical well-being. Parkes (1972) reported more bereaved patients in a psychiatric population than should have been present by chance. Connolly (1975) showed that widowers over 55 years of age have mortality rates above the expected rate for age-matched married men and identified a period, six months after bereavement, as being a vulnerable time. Parkes reported that there was little evidence of planning for the future in two-thirds of the widows studied at the end of the first year. The bereaved would often show little interest in food, sleep, or personal appearance. There are direct parallels with the apathy which develops in the infant deprived of contact with its mother for a long period.

When we examine the possible basis of the response to loss there are two possibilities. The first is that the response patterns could be organised biologically. In other words there might be 'loss detectors' in the nervous system which trigger early panic and high anxiety states and mobilise searching behaviour. Good reason could be provided for such an automatic system. It would be of evolutionary advantage for the response to loss to be fast and appropriate. Searching, striving and obvious distress are perhaps the best way of attracting the parent or other help in the young infant.

The medical model of bereavement was proposed by Lindemann (1944) who likened the associated biological and behavioural responses to symptoms and referred to grief as a syndrome. In spite of this approach, Lindemann produced little by way of a clear account of how the bereavement 'disease' might be orchestrated.

A second possibility is that the response pattern is cognitively determined. The appraisal of loss would be assumed to lead to perceived threat, and cause the implementation of plans for fighting or fleeing, resulting in raised levels of arousal.

Figure 2.1 (from Fisher, 1984) illustrates a possible conceptualisation of understanding the reaction to loss. The model is capable of providing a biological or a cognitive basis for understanding the response to loss. It is based on the principles of Von Holst's model of reafference (Von Holst, 1954) and ideomotor theory (see Greenwald, 1970). The basic assumption of the model is simple: when actions are produced (see A in Fig. 2.1), *copies* of each action are stored in the nervous system (see AC in Fig. 2.1) Each copy (AC) is associated in memory with expectancies (AE) about likely consequences indicated by action-produced feedback (AF). If the consequence of action is unexpected, then the signals in the comparator are discrepant (AE/AF mismatch) and there is potential input to an alarm system with implication for raised arousal and anxious behaviour. As shown in Fig. 2.1 the potential input to the alarm system is first subject to a cost evaluation system which decides how important is the discrepancy.

In terms of a concrete example, a young infant responds to its mother and has expectancies about the consequences of action. If the mother fails to respond appropriately, or is absent, the consequence as perceived by the infant will be discrepant with what was expected. The mismatch between

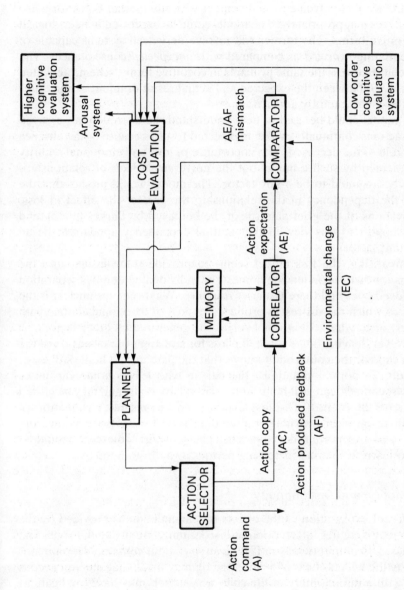

FIG. 2.1. Representation of processes in the perception of control as a function of personal influence—based on ideomotor theory (Fisher, 1984).

what the infant expected and what happened should result in an increase in alarm accompanied by anxious striving behaviour. The model assumes that loss of control is perceived when contact with the mother is lost or when she behaves inappropriately. The model could be expressed in neurological or cognitive terms. The former will involve nerve-cell systems capable of differentiating *expected* as compared with *unexpected* consequences. The latter could express the same principle in cognitive terms; schema activated by *mismatch* between the expected and actual result of infant action differ from those activated by a *match*.

The model could be used to help understand the distress of a bereaved adult; actions continually evoke unexpected results because of the absence of the role of the deceased. The importance of love and emotional security is not denied by such a model but the nurturant aspects of relationships would be assumed to be a key factor. The model would predict that the closer the dependency in the relationship the greater the effect of loss. Observations of the grief patterns of the bereaved by Parkes (1972) lend some support to this view in that mutual dependency appears to be an important factor.

Summarising, the loss model seems to provide some insight into the reasons for distress on leaving home. The individual undergoes separation from loved ones and there is a grief response. What remains unclear is the extent to which the distress is produced by loss of emotional contact with parents, or to what extent it is likely to be generated by other factors.

However, leaving home is not like loss for a number of reasons. First the grown child or the young adult knows that the parents and home still exist. Secondly, in normal situations, the person who leaves home can make symbolic contact, can visit home at prescribed intervals, and may be visited by parents or friends. The loss experienced, represents termination of immediate physical proximity rather than total loss. Also moving from home is part of normal development. The growing adolescent should be able to learn to tolerate increasing periods away from home.

Interruption and Discontinuity

A different explanation of the effects of leaving home is provided by the notion that it creates interruption or discontinuity in existing life-styles and routines. Discontinuity may in fact be an important common denominator of many life events. Loss of a close person may mean that the bereaved is faced with a discontinuity in life-style which itself may have implications for psychological and physical health. The widow has to learn to deal with situations previously coped with by the deceased, etc.

Laboratory studies involving the contrived interruption of tasks (see

Mandler, 1975) have provided a great deal of evidence to suggest that a likely effect is increased arousal, manifest as anxiety in some cases. Mandler and Watson (1966) demonstrated that interruption of an on-going laboratory task will result in persistence towards completion of the interrupted sequence; increased vigour with which the sequence is pursued, and attempts to substitute alternative elements or sequences. Interruption of existing routines following a move is very different from interruption of laboratory tasks but there may be properties in common. Perhaps plans which previously dominate behaviour continue to dominate, and drive inappropriate thoughts or activities in the new environment. Thus the domination and persistence of old plans might be partly responsible for the reactions to leaving home. Nostalgia (derived from 'nosos' meaning past and 'algia' meaning pain) might be triggered and maintained by specific functional attributes of the organisation of planning. The capacity of plans to dominate attention and when inappropriate, to create an inefficient state of mental function in relation to the new environment, may well have origins in evolutionary survival. Fisher (1984) notes that reflective activity involving past plans might be a prerequisite for the development of new effective plans. The process might be fundamental in allowing acquired resources from previous experience to be integrated into future plans.

It is also conceivable that the sense of separation and loss is triggered by the dominance of old plans in memory. The individual cannot help thinking about home because old plans (ways of going into a room, cooking a meal, or taking a bath) come readily to mind. To illustrate this with respect to the example of trying to give up eating chocolate bars; the individual faced with reminders such as pictures of chocolate etc. might find it more difficult; the stimuli act as prompts. Perhaps planned activity is so structured that dominant old plans persist and can prompt imagined scenarios.

The Control Model

The control model offers an explanation which can only be understood in terms of the general theory of stress and its effects on behaviour. Increasingly, definitions of stress have emphasised the importance of the interaction of the individual with the environment. Stress is often not 'out there' in the world but is in part created by properties of the structure of cognition in individuals (see Fisher, 1984; 1986).

The concept of control or power and mastery of the environment, fits within this framework. Increasingly there has been research interest in the notion that when control is possible because of instrumentality or skill, then threatening events become less so. Some backing for these ideas has come from the animal studies where being given the means to escape shock creates less extensive ulceration or weight loss than being helpless (see Mowrer & Viek, 1948; Weiss, 1968; 1970).

Studies with human beings are rather less convincing in that for example, self-administration of shock, although likely to be chosen by about two-thirds of a population, is less likely to create changes in the physiological repsonse to shock than to tolerance, or judgements about level of anxiety (see Fisher, 1986; 1988b). Also, in the case of human beings it seems that control may be relinquished to 'powerful others' as when a person consults a dentist or medical practitioner. Fisher (1986) argues that in such cases control may be exercised via the inter-personal domain, in that the act of choice (to visit a dentist) is itself a form of control in order to achieve the best final product (painless tooth removal).

Fisher (1986) provided a decision model of control in which three domains of control were identified—personal, inter-personal and socio-political. In each domain, a person makes a decision as to whether or not control facility is available, and whether or not the skilled resource exists. Thus as illustrated by Fig. 2.2, the individual who leaves home might be engaged in quite complex decision-making about the world he confronts.

In spite of many of the difficulties outlined above, loss of control is cited frequently as a likely common denominator of different life threats and outcomes. It is frequently seen to have properties in common with help-lessness and depression. Loss of control in a threatening situation can also be a precurser of illness because of the likelihood of the production of hormones which suppress the immune response (Fisher, 1988a; 1988b). Control has been identified by Karasek (1979) as an important determinant of job strain. From the results of an analysis of the stress levels of Swedish and American workers, Karasek argues that job strain occurs when demand is high but discretionality or jurisdiction is low. A sense of challenge and positive stress is greater when demand is high but discretionality is high. This is the condition experienced by executives and managers.

Fisher (1986) developed the control theory of the response to change and transition arguing that many major life events including a move away from home result in a period of reduction of control. New aspects of life have to be learned and new skills acquired. The widow must learn for example to cope with running the household without help normally given by the spouse. The person who moves needs to learn about a new location, new faces, new routines etc. Precisely because the environment is new, there will be less control initially. There is in effect a step function change in the world. Obtaining control means acquiring skills and learning about instrumental features of the environment (where to park the car; where to find a bank; how to cope with shopping hours; the new population, etc). Thus change may not itself be threatening *per se*. In fact people choose

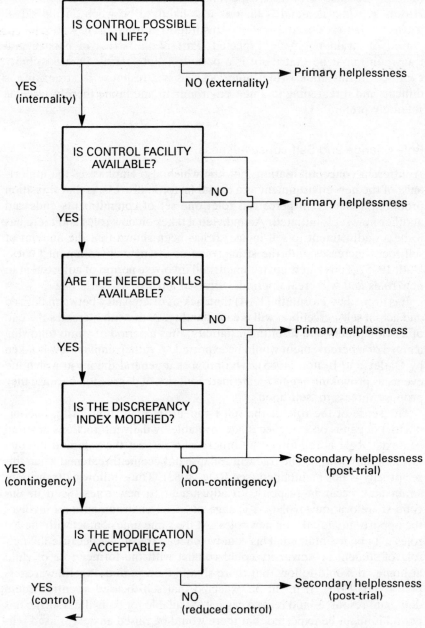

FIG. 2.2.   Hierarchically ordered decisions in the perception of control in specific situations (Fisher, 1986).

holidays because they can experience new, stimulating environments. However, when demand is high as it is likely to be when an individual leaves home to reside at a school or institution or to take a new job, then a period of strain might be expected. Part of the stress of change and transition might be that there is a period of 'job strain'. One possibility explored in this book is that homesickness is a response to strain; life is difficult and threatening in a new environment and home therefore seems infinitely preferable.

Role Change and Self-consciousness

A different conceptualisation, but one which also emphasises the importance of the new environment as a causal factor in distress, is that transition produces a change in perceived role; one set of commitments ends and another new set is initiated. An individual takes on new roles and there has to be an adjustment to self-image. It has been shown that the amount of self-focus increases with the strangeness of the new environment (Wickland, 1975). Thus a new environment will involve a period of adjustment to new roles and will create periods of raised anxiety.

It is argued by Hormuth (1984) that lack of discrepancy between desired and actual self-perception will create stability. A transition creates the end of a commitment and resulting instability; thus a period of strain following a move or a bereavement would be expected. A rather similar view is taken by Oatley and Bolton (1985), who propose a general theory in which life events as provoking agents create increased risk of depression because they propose threats to 'self-hood'.

The sense of the role of the self (student; mother; housewife; banker; doctor) depends on evidence made available by daily interactions in social contexts. Role is reinforced by others who respect the role and interact meaningfully with it. The role will collapse or become threatened when this reciprocity is not maintained (see Ryle, 1982). Thus, following transition, strain may occur in response to adjustment to new roles. Seen in this context, relocation involves a change of social environment and involves the opportunity to take on new roles. At the same time contact with the old roles may be maintained. This could even lead to conflict because the new role of student at university could conflict with the former role of child at home. It would follow that there should be a period of self-awareness (Wickland, 1975). It might be expected that self-focused attention could dominate resources and reduce capacity available for daily life. During this period it might be expected that there would be raised anxiety, raised self-preoccupation and perhaps for that reason raised absent-mindedness. These aspects would reflect in distress and the systems which characterise distress.

The Effects of Conflict

One possibility which must also be considered, is that a person opts to give up security and comfort associated with life at home in order to obtain new experiences, social, educational or financial improvements. For some people this may create a conflict; home is more secure and the new environment is less secure but more challenging. The conflict might be particularly evident for university or medical school students where obtaining a place is a privilege and the conflict between wanting to persist with such an educational opportunity and yet return home could be great. By comparison, nursing training may produce less of a conflict because the alternative possibilities are greater for nurses to live near home and gain work in hospitals.

Cameron and Margaret (1951) gave central importance to conflict as a causal factor in psychopathology. They noted the prevalence of conflict in clinical groups and identified different conflict typologies based on approach and avoidance elements. Homesickness might be part of an approach-avoidance conflict in which the new environment creates both approach and avoidant tendencies. If conflict exists then we might expect individuals to be mentally preoccupied with considering the conflicting decisions. This should result in raised absent-mindedness.

SUMMARY AND CONCLUSIONS

On first consideration, there are a number of reasons why the transition from home to take up residence in a new environment, should be distressing. There is immediate loss of physical proximity with family and friends, interruption of routines and habits, a likely change in role; a step function change in the new environment and the loss of loved security and comforts.

In this chapter we have reviewed five theoretical models which provide a basis for understanding the distress evident for some of those who leave home.

The loss model suggests that there might be a grief-like response characterised by anxious searching behaviour and panic. The individual in effect is experiencing a mini-bereavement. The only difference is of course that the loss is reversible and contact with loved ones and home can be maintained.

Interruption theory would also predict raised anxiety because of the effects of the termination of previous habits and routines. If substitute activities are not found, anxiety levels could remain high.

The control model predicts raised depression because in the new environment there is lack of knowledge about routines and procedures. The period of loss of control should result in depression. Thus we would expect changes towards raised depression following the move from home.

The role model again places emphasis on the new environment but assumes that there would be raised anxiety and self-preoccupation due to the demands of new roles. We would expect raised anxiety and perhaps absent-mindedness to be symptomatic.

Finally we have identified a conflict model in which the security of home is balanced against the insecurity, but also the challenge and interest of the new environment. The individual may experience the conflict of wanting to go home where it is secure and comfortable, but feel the challenge of the opportunities provided by the new environment. Such a conflict could produce high states of anxiety.

It is unlikely that these theoretical models can be distinguished in terms of ability to predict the manifestations of stress following the transition from home. However, there is some indication that we might expect to find raised anxiety (loss model, interruption model, role model, conflict model) and raised depression (control model). All the theories imply that there will be reason for reflective activity and self-preoccupation; such states should create periods of absent-mindedness.

3

The Incidence and Features of Homesickness

'Homesickness' is a term which exists in many languages and is used to describe the psychological experiences which occur following a transition. It is particularly pertinent for situations where a person leaves home, including family and friends, to take up residence in another location. Most typically this involves young people who leave home for educational, training or vocational purposes. In the U.K, children as young as seven may leave home to attend a primary school as boarders. This is particularly likely for those in the upper socio-economic income brackets. Children are sent away to school as part of a privileged educational system, although, children may also be sent away from home if they commit crimes or petty offences. The majority of children who leave home for boarding school are between 11 and 13 years old and do so for their secondary education.

DEFINITIONS AND CORRELATES OF HOMESICKNESS

Homesickness is commonly described in terms of antecedents such as 'missing home' *(Chambers Twentieth Century Dictionary)*. Some definitions include symptoms as well. For example, a common definition is 'depressed by absence from home' *(Concise Oxford English Dictionary)*. The implication is that a person yearns for, or grieves for, the former (home) environment and becomes depressed as a result.

Those who work in an administrative, counselling or a care capacity in schools and universities frequently use the term 'homesickness' to describe the distress experience observed in many of those students who arrive for the first time. However, there has been no formal recognition of the term

21

to describe either a clinical or a non-clinical condition. The issue concerning the role of the homesickness response as part of the process of adaptation to transitions has not been considered.

Research on homesickness involves a number of problems relating to the lack of formal or clinical classification and diagnosis. Homesickness is similar to grief in that it seems to be a very specific manifestation of distress associated with a known cause. However severe the grief response is, it tends to be regarded as non-clinical because it is part of a normal response to bereavement. In fact the grief pattern is subject to cultural rules and social expectations. Although the victim of grief is treated with caution, the condition is respected and seen to be normal by others. Only when grief reactions are protracted or the expression of the emotion is impaired, is the condition considered to have pathological properties.

Lindemann (1944) tried to work with a medical model of the grief response pattern. Implicit in the approach is that the grief is a syndrome (linked collection of symptoms) with an organic cause. Lindemann, however, failed to justify this position; his own therapeutic technique involved psychological manipulations.

It appears that in the case of both the grief and homesickness reaction patterns, a single psychogenic factor (life event), the properties of which are known, can precipitate the experience of a distress reaction which is engineered within the constraint of the operation of normal mechanisms. Thus the grief and homesickness response patterns could be regarded as distress reactions which have common features. The differentiating factors are the cognitive orientations which specifically reflect the psychogenic factor regarded as the cause. If, for example, a person who was bereaved was in one room and a person who was homesick was in another, and the job of the investigator was to decide which person was homesick and which was bereaved by asking only one question, that question should concern the focus of cognitive activity and not the nature of the distress symptoms.

One possibility is that both grief and homesickness are forms of reactive depression which could be clinical in some cases and which differ in cognitive aspects from other forms of depression. Thus depression characterised by a pervading sense of loss is distinguished from forms of depression characterised by for example failure.

A common denominator central to depressed mood may be loss of control. The homesick person desires to (but cannot) restore the daily experience of being at home; the bereaved cannot restore the experience of being with the deceased; in circumstances of failure a particular aim is thwarted. On the above analysis it is the lack of ability to reverse the situation that is the common denominator which leads to depression.

One of the difficulties with understanding the effects of leaving home on mental health is that the nature of the circumstances surrounding the move may vary greatly. Wapner et al. (1981) recognise 'critical transitions' which disrupt equilibrium, as compared with transitions which really represent a smooth on-going set of plans. Enforced disruptions produced by pressure to move would create conditions of critical transitions. They argue that although not all critical transitions lead to disruptions, many create a sense of overwhelming loss and change the self-world relationship. Thus in trying to assess the likely influence of leaving home on mental state, it is necessary not just to consider the process of transition but the *background* against which it occurs and the pressures which might force a conflict between leaving or staying at home. Equally, it is necessary to consider the stage in a person's life at which a particular transition occurs.

EARLY WORK ON HOMESICKNESS

The importance of homesickness as a factor in health and well-being is underlined by early medical interest in the topic. An early treatise in the form of a medical text (Harder, 1678) refers to the adverse experience of adults experiencing a relocation in terms of 'maladie du pays'. The term 'nostalgia' was also introduced to describe the experience; the derivation is 'nostos' which is Greek for return home and 'algos' meaning 'pain or sorrow'. Harder believed that a number of remote or predisposing causes create in the mind strong thoughts of returning home. The antecedent causes were assumed to be differences in habits, food and customs, together with insults and injuries. By contrast, Zuckert (1768) provided an explanation of homesickness observed in his patients, which he assumed to be related to their illness symptoms. He argued that the emotional stability of the person was the critical factor. Thus from 17th and 18th century medical writings the contrasting notions of internal *'vulnerability'* factors as compared with *external cause* are emphasised. If a relocation is assumed to be a necessary condition for homesickness, it clearly cannot from these early writings be a sufficient condition. The emphasis focuses on circumstantial and personal determinants (see Chapter 2).

The importance of the homesickness reaction in accounting for somatic symptoms and illness was underlined by Corp (1791) in a study of relocations in British Army recruits. The symptoms observed in one recruit were giddiness, noise in the ears, bad dreams, insomnia, and melancholy. The patient was described as 'wasting away'. The condition improved on returning home.

Peacock (1988) quotes Tausk (1969) who as physician of the Austrian Army highlighted the significance of homesickness as a major cause of desertion during the First World War. When the situation is unpleasant in battle, there may be signs of escape into reveries and fantasy. This may be a precurser of the escape from reality in order to return home. Tausk identified cognitive, affective and motivational components of the condition. Principle features included loss of control, loneliness and abandonment, plus preparation for returning home (flight). He also noted the link with 'solitude psychosis'.

In spite of early medical interest, there has been little by way of systematic research, but there have been a number of studies which describe the phenomenon. Hojat and Herman (1985) investigated the adjustment to American culture in foreign medical graduates and note the difficulties in communication and interpersonal relations which lead to feelings of alienation and a wish to return home. They report a relationship with homesickness and low self-esteem and note that it was frequent in Filipino physicians.

Nicassio and Pate (1984) reported that over half of a sample of Indo-Chinese refugees experienced homesickness. Separation from family, loneliness, and communication problems with home, were combined with memories of the unpleasant effects of war. All these may have collectively influenced adjustment and were assumed to be causal factors in the homesickness experience.

Studies of the adaptation to migration frequently emphasise the homesickness response, however there is very little in-depth analysis of what the term means to individuals and how it is to be assessed. The association with personal grief for loss of friends and family and personal loneliness is emphasised. Some investigators do not distinguish the homesickness response from a general grief reaction (e.g., see Arrendondo-Dowd, 1981).

A cursory analysis of homesickness was provided as part of a study by Torbjorn (1982), who in an investigation of the adaptation of Swedes to living abroad, included two statements which he argued assessed homesickness. The first was 'Sweden is a country to return to in old age'; the second was 'After some time abroad one does not miss Sweden any more' (p. 113). Torbjorn argued that acute homesickness was indicated if there was an answer of 'fully agree' to the first question and 'disagree entirely' to the second question. Answers to the first question suggested an incidence level of 30% whereas answers to the second question indicated an incidence level of 20%. The correlation between responses on the two questions was 0.33 (no significance level indicated). Unfortunately this investigation could hardly be described as thorough and it is not clear to what extent the fundamental aspects of homesickness were being tapped by these questions. Many people might want to return home as they grow old for all kinds of practical reasons.

THE INCIDENCE OF HOMESICKNESS

The Semantics of Homesickness

In this section we consider some of the features of homesickness incidence. In investigating the factors affecting incidence, we found many of the problems which remain unsolved issues in the diagnosis of clinical states. Do people know what is wrong, given that they feel disturbed or unhappy? If not can they answer questions about symptoms in order that a skilled expert can reach an overall diagnosis? These problems seem to involve the same issue. If it is not reasonable to ask a person 'are you depressed', is it reasonable to ask questions such as 'are you often unhappy for no good reason'. Do victims of experience label and describe the experience clearly? Do victims of an experience use an available label to describe it more readily than they do spontaneously generate it? Do victims who have an experience use the term in the same way as those who have never had the experience? We might expect a sufferer with back-ache to find more features with which to describe back-ache than a non-sufferer. These and many related issues formed the focus for many protracted discussions. The solution ended up as a compromise between the ideal and the possible, but at least some attempt was made to explore the underlying issues.

The 'Labelling' Problem. Individuals may be more tempted to use a prompted question or label to describe their experiences, but less likely to think of using the term spontaneously. This is an important issue because all questionnaire and diagnostic tests which depend on self-report involve this difficulty. If a person is more likely to say that he or she is depressed when the term is provided for endorsement, as compared with free recall in the absence of all prompts, then the presentation mode is the critical factor and report incidence will be unstable. Most assessments of incidence of psychological states depend on recognition rather than recall, or involve classification of recalled 'symptoms' by experts (psychiatrists, clinical psychologists, etc.).

A study by Fisher, Frazer, and Murray (1984) showed that when the term 'homesickness' was not mentioned and boarding school pupils merely provided daily information about problems and worries on arrival at a new school, the spontaneous incidence of homesickness was only 18%. However, if the term was made available for endorsement the incidence was much higher: 60–70% of first-year students and boarding school pupils report the experience on arrival for the first time in residence at University or boarding school respectively (see Fisher et al., 1985, 1986). Thus, the presentation mode may have a very important effect on reported incidence. Perhaps when the label is present for endorsement it acts as a catalyst for the grouping of feelings of distress.

When names of subjects are required, the tendency to report homesickness is lower. Thus the willingness to use an available term depends on other situational factors as well as portrayal of the self. As will be indicated later, there is some evidence that homesickness is not socially sanctioned and that the victim of the experience feels 'wimpish' if he reports it. This is a very important issue for counsellors and general practitioners, because it may account for occasions when patients report with pseudo-symptoms but eventually introduce the real problem.

The issue may also be important because individuals of, for example, low self-esteem may be more willing to report an experience even though it is not socially sanctioned. This would mean that population differences may reflect the operation of a hidden variable which determines reporting bias.

There are special difficulties with experiences which involve adaptation following a life event. The experience is 'state' rather than 'trait' and will change with time. Thus, the occasion when assessment is obtained may be a critical factor in determining incidence.

The Problem of Social Desirability. As already described there is evidence to suggest that homesickness is not socially sanctioned in response to a life event in the way that bereavement is.

Some illustration that the experience of homesickness is socially undesirable has come from the results of a study in which 68 university students were provided with a brief description of a (hypothetical) student and were asked to rate that student's expected quality on a number of attributes on a five point scale from nought (most negative) to five (most positive). There were three judgement groups. The first group of 21 judges were given a description of a student which included the statement that he experienced homesickness when leaving home. The second group of 22 judges were given a description of a student which included the statement that he had experienced the distress of bereavement when a relative died. The third group of 25 judges were given no information at all about homesickness or bereavement (control condition). As illustrated in Table 3.1, the presence of information indicating that the hypothetical person had been homesick,

TABLE 3.1

Pilot Study of Attitudes to Homesickness Based on Judgements of a
Hypothetical Person Described as 'Homesick' (in press)

Alleged Attributes for Hypothetical Person (Rated Qualities on a 5-point Scale)	Homesick		Not Homesick		Control		Kruskal Wallis ANOVA p Values
	$\bar{\chi}$	SD	$\bar{\chi}$	SD	$\bar{\chi}$	SD	
Intelligence (0–5)	3.1	0.9	4.2	1.8	3.9	1.1	$0.01 > p > 0.001$
Friendships (0–5)	2.0	1.1	3.9	1.3	4.1	1.0	$0.02 > p > 0.01$
Success at University (0–5)	2.9	1.3	3.8	1.2	3.7	0.8	$0.01 > p > 0.001$

lowered the judgements of levels of success, intelligence, and social desirability.

These data are important in indicating the lack of social recognition of homesickness as either a clinical state or a 'reasonable' psychological experience requiring guidance and surveillance. This fits with observations made by sufferers; it is often remarked by those who are homesick that it is childish or silly to be homesick. If society has been slow to recognise the importance of the profound and uncontrollable effects of bereavement, in spite of adverse behavioural and health consequences with which it is associated, it has been negligent in developing any understanding of the importance of homesickness and distress which may follow transitions from home. It is left to sufferers to self-select help from counsellors, colleagues or other authorities and yet help-seeking may itself be prevented by the withdrawal characteristics associated with the condition.

Unlike bereavement, the homesickness experience is self-limiting in that the sufferer could go home. However, as argued previously, the conflict between fulfilling personal and parental ambition may be very strong and giving up may itself be associated with distress because of perceived failure to take advantage of opportunities for educational and vocational advancement over a 'trivial' phenomenon.

Much of what has been discussed above is illustrated by the content of letters sent to the research unit during the period of the research, following press publicity:

Thank God, someone has made this a respectable topic for study. I spent about 10 years of my young adult life away from home at university and training college in a state of abject misery and grief. I cried quietly at nights, dreading the fact that someone would find out. People who knew me thought of me as 'depressed' and I suppose I was, but there was a reason for my depression that I couldn't reveal—I wanted to go home so badly it was intolerable. Worse, I could not tell my parents, I had to pretend I was happy . . . (Male, age 35)

I was sick, dazed, ill, unable to cope and ashamed of my constant grief for home. I spent all day imagining what I would be doing if I was at home. I couldn't eat properly. I stopped going out to lectures after the first week. I just lay about in my room lost in thought and swamped with unhappiness. I lived in dread that everyone else would find out. I made no friends . . . (Female, age 27)

The noise and people overwhelmed me. I was ill but did not know why I was ill. I wanted to ring my parents and friends up. I wrote hundreds of letters. I contemplated suicide. I couldn't cope with the work. I became ashamed of my own state—I thought I must be weak because no-one else seemed worried . . . (Female, age 24)

Recording the Incidence and Level of Homesickness

The above section was concerned with depicting in general terms the difficulties of studying an intense, distressing experience which is generally regarded as non-clinical, which if anything is not socially acceptable as an experience, and which may even be perceived (by sufferers or non-sufferers) as a sign of weakness.

To attempt to investigate homesickness means starting from the very beginning and trying to describe the boundaries of the experience. There are no clinical experts who could provide diagnostic criteria and very little indication of how the condition might relate to state/trait issues or to clinical states. Self-report of the state of homesickness was the only means of assessment which was possible. As already described, provision of the term may precipitate the reporting of homesickness. It was also possible that recording format and style of report required continued to be influential.

A series of three different diary-style formats for obtaining records of experiences in the first two weeks of new school or university term were designed. The school version was designed for use in local boarding school by pupils of 11 years old or over and contained explicit instructions with illustrations of how to fill in the diary and how to present an indication of personal life history. The same format was used for the students, but the instructions were presented in a more mature form.

Figure 3.1 illustrates a version of the diary format where up to 4 problems could be reported and a column labelled 'periods of homesickness' enabled the subject to report homesickness. There were 3 versions of the diary format. The first did not include the 'homesickness' column but is otherwise identical to the illustrated format in Fig. 3.1. The second version is represented in Fig. 3.1. The third version is devoted totally to questions about homesickness.

Columns in each diary format are drawn up against a time scale representing the hours of the day. Instructions indicate that on each day a person can identify up to 4 problems (or no problems) and allocate each problem to a column by describing it underneath the appropriate column. Against the time scale representing a 12-hour day for boarding school pupils (night hours were not included in case it encouraged loss of sleep) and 24 hours for students, a respondent could indicate periods of worry and preoccupation with a particular problem. This provides an index of how often a person could remember worrying about a problem. The first version of the diary enables us to obtain an index of how often homesickness is spontaneously reported by pupils or students in the first two weeks of the new school or university term.

Unfortunately, although the school returns were successful (100%) the

TODAY'S DATE 4/10/83

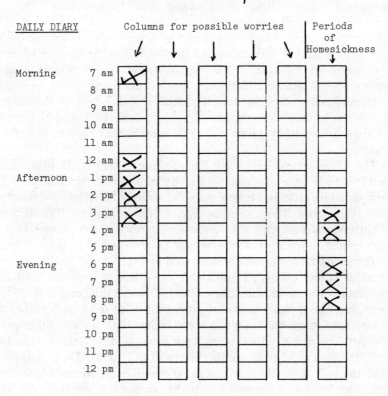

FIG. 3.1. Example of diary record for one out of the first fourteen days, from a first-year university student.

student returns (20–30%) were not high enough to enable valid conclusions to be drawn. The school returns were high because although the diaries were completed anonymously, the system ensured that each pupil handed in a diary. The problem with sampling university students in this way is that there is little incentive for them to make anonymous returns. Perhaps more importantly, the start of a new university term means that most students receive a plethora of leaflets and information regarding the university and its clubs and societies. Student welfare groups solicit opinions on aspects of union and student life. Against this background, completion of two-week diaries is probably too demanding and diaries are likely to be lost.

The school return for the first diary format (Fisher et al., 1984) indicated that there was 16% spontaneous use of the term homesickness in 50 diaries completed by male and female pupils in a mixed sex (female minority) city boarding school. There were no age or sex differences. The data on the occurrence of problems with associated periods of worry, provided some very useful information which we will be referring to in later chapters.

The second diary format is illustrated by Fig. 3.1 and provided a column headed 'homesickness'; respondents were free to endorse cells in that column in order to indicate homesickness. Under this condition, 76% of 17 boarding school pupils provided an indication of the experience of homesickness. Homesickness reports were higher than for any other problem category: there was a total of 90 reports across all subjects for the 14 days and 201 associated worry units (Fisher et al., 1986). These data indicate that there is a labelling problem; there is a difference of 18–20% in incidence level as a function of whether or not the question is prompted.

The third diary format focused entirely on homesickness. The diary was so arranged that subjects indicated for each day whether or not homesickness had been reported and by means of endorsements in columns, what social and behavioural conditions were present at the time. The reported incidence of homesickness was 71% for 21 pupils (Fisher et al., 1986).

In later studies with students, five category rating scales based on self-reported frequency of homesickness were used (see Fisher et al., 1985). The use of frequency scales did not influence the incidence levels of self-reported homesickness. Taken collectively these data indicate that although, as previously described, there is a labelling problem, further manipulations of format for response make little difference.

Personal Meanings of the Term 'Homesickness'

One very important prerequisite for all the self-report studies carried out is that there is an indication of each person's understanding of the meaning of the term 'homesickness' and that sufferers and non-sufferers use the term in the same way. Perhaps, as already argued, sufferers of any condition whether it is psychological or physical, learn more about the experience. For example, a person who has experienced a painful back may be expected to give a more detailed account of what 'back-ache' means.

All subjects who took part in the studies were rountinely asked to provide a written definition of the term 'homesick'. Table 3.2(a) and (b) provide an indication of key features of the term as classified from the results of a study with students (Fisher et al., 1985) and with boarding school children (Fisher et at., 1986). The definitions provided varied in length and content. Some individuals provided very long definitions such as 'missing home, parents, and friends and wishing you had never left home'; 'crying because I want to go home to my family because I miss them and I hate it here'. Some definitions were academic; 'missing home'; 'grieving for home'. Others indicated symptoms; 'missing home so much you cry and feel sick and cannot sleep'.

Each description was partitioned into elements and then each element classified. This was carried out with all investigators present. There was no initial structure, each set of definitions provided the basis for evolving the classification. Data such as these cannot be used for analytic procedures since the boundary of each grouping is a variable and will differ in size. Thus 'missing home, family and friends' could be partitioned into 'missing home', 'missing family', 'missing friends'. Alternatively, these elements could be regarded as part of a total 'home' concept and grouped together. Different agreed criteria create different cells and therefore cells vary in size and thus in the frequency of associated entries.

The two selected tables show that the greatest frequency of elements in the definitions concern missing parents/home environment and friends. However, the data also indicate that definitions from boarding school pupils (aged 11–14) contain a greater frequency of elements concerned with parents and family (65.9% and 75.8% for homesick and non-homesick children respectively), as compared with students where these elements occurred less frequently (33.3% and 30.0% for homesick and non-homesick students respectively). Therefore, the focus of the themes in the definitions may reflect age differences. This has not been specifically investigated partly because of the unavoidable methodological difficulties described above.

The tables also indicate that whilst there are dominant themes in the definitions concerned with the antecedent condition 'missing home' etc., there are also symptoms and attitudes to the new institution. For example, there are 'orientation' elements—'feeling lost'; 'feeling disoriented'. There are elements which are motivational and express mood state—feeling unhappy, dissatisfied, emotional, depressed, sad, anxious and tearful.

Generally, homesickness appears to be a complex cognitive-motivational-emotional state focused on missing home. The symptoms included vary between individuals and may reflect personal reactions to distress or

TABLE 3.2(a)
Features Utilised in Definitions of Homesickness for Homesick and
Non-homesick First-year Students

Feature Categories From Definitions Provided	Frequency of Reported Features and Percentage of Subjects Reporting Each Feature	
	Homesick (n = 60) f(%)	Non-homesick (n = 60) f(%)
'Missing home environment'; 'Missing house, home, area etc.'	18 (30.0)	16 (40.0)
'Missing parents/family'; 'Longing for people at home'	20 (33.3)	12 (30.0)
'Wanting to go home'; 'Feeling a need to return home'	14 (23.3)	11 (27.5)
'Missing friends'; 'Longing for friends'	18 (30.0)	5 (12.5)
'Feeling of loneliness'	3 (5.0)	7 (17.5)
'Feeling depressed'	3 (5.0)	3 (7.5)
'Missing someone close to talk to'	4 (6.7)	1 (2.5)
'Feeling insecure'	3 (5.0)	2 (5.0)
'Obsession with thoughts of home'; 'Thoughts about home'	3 (5.0)	3 (7.5)
'Feeling unhappy'	1 (1.7)	3 (7.5)
'Feeling unloved'	2 (3.3)	1 (2.5)
'Disorientation'; 'Feeling lost in new environment'	2 (3.3)	1 (2.5)
'A longing for familiar company and places'	1 (1.7)	1 (2.5)
'Thinking of the past'	1 (1.7)	2 (5.0)
'Feeling of not belonging'	1 (1.7)	1 (2.5)
'Regret that life had changed'; 'A feeling of regret'	3 (5.0)	0 (0.0)
'Feeling isolated'; 'Cut off from the world'	2 (3.3)	1 (2.5)
'Feeling uneasy'	0 (0.0)	2 (5.0)
'Feeling ill'	1 (1.7)	0 (0.0)
'Dissatisfaction with present situation'	1 (1.7)	0 (0.0)
'Unable to cope'	1 (1.7)	0 (0.0)
'Unable to do anything'	1 (1.7)	0 (0.0)
'Hating the present place'	0 (0.0)	1 (2.5)

NOTE: The following features were endorsed by only one person in the following groups. Homesick: 'Thinking that home was better than here'; 'Feeling of making a mistake'; 'Sinking feeling in stomach'; 'Loss of appetite'; 'Feeling of desperation' and 'Crying'. Non-homesick: 'New self-reliance'; 'Feeling of desolation' and 'Feeling unsettled'.

SOURCE: Fisher, Murray, and Frazer (1985).

TABLE 3.2(b)
Features Utilised in Definitions of Homesickness for Homesick and
Non-homesick School Pupils

Feature Categories From Definitions Provided	Frequency of Reported Features and Percentage of Subjects Reporting Each Feature	
	Homesick (n = 82) f(%)	Non-homesick (n = 33) f(%)
'Missing parent family'; 'longing for people at home'	54 (65.9)	25 (75.8)
'Missing home environment'; 'missing house, home, area, etc.'	28 (34.1)	12 (36.4)
'Wanting to go home'; 'feeling a need to return home'	21 (25.6)	10 (30.3)
'Missing friends'; 'longing for friends'	12 (14.6)	1 (3.0)
'Feeling of loneliness'	10 (12.2)	1 (3.0)
'Crying'	3 (3.7)	3 (9.1)
'Unsettled'	4 (4.9)	1 (3.0)
'Hating the present place'	4 (4.9)	1 (3.0)
'Feeling unhappy'	4 (4.9)	1 (3.0)
'Not getting on with people'	3 (3.7)	0 (0.0)
'Dissatisfaction with present situation'	3 (3.7)	0 (0.0)
'Feeling depressed'	2 (2.4)	1 (3.0)
'Disorientation'; 'feeling lost in new environment'	2 (2.4)	0 (0.0)
'Regret that life had changed', 'A feeling of regret'	2 (2.4)	0 (0.0)
'Never been away from home before'	2 (2.4)	0 (0.0)
'Feeling ill'	2 (2.4)	0 (0.0)
'Unable to do anything'	2 (2.4)	0 (0.0)
'Feeling unloved'	0 (0.0)	2 (6.1)

NOTE: The following features were endorsed by only one person in the following groups. *Homesick*: 'problem at school'; 'missing someone close to talk to'; 'obsession with thoughts of home'; 'looking for familiar company and faces'; 'feeling isolated'. *Non-homesick*: 'feeling uneasy'; 'unable to cope'; 'feeling full and weary'; 'thinking home is better than here'.
SOURCE: Fisher, Frazer, and Murray (1986).

personal perceptions of the threat the transition creates. Fortunately, in all studies reported, the definitions of homesickness provided by respondents did not distinguish those who reported experiencing homesickness and those who did not, either in terms of the number of reported elements (i.e. length/complexity or definition) or in terms of rank order or frequency of elements. There were positive correlations of 0.65–0.91 on a non-parametic ranking test (Spearman's correlation) between the frequencies of elements in definitions given by those who reported homesick experiences and those who reported no homesickness. Thus, we can be reasonably satisfied that subjects are using the term in a way which concords with other subjects, irrespective of whether or not they are homesickness reporters.

THE CHARACTERISTICS OF HOMESICKNESS INCIDENCE

As already indicated, homesickness reporting is influenced by whether or not the label is available for endorsement. After that it seems not to matter how the term is presented or what sort of recording format is used.

Definitions of the term did not distinguish the homesick from the non-homesick. It seems that all subjects focus primarily on missing and grieving for home/family and friends as the main feature. This is fortunate in enabling us to equate the homesick and non-homesick subjects because of concordance in the use of the term.

In the U.K. studies, a stable 60–70% incidence of homesickness report-ing was obtained across all subject groups except when names of subjects were obtained for identification purposes in longitudinal studies. Incidence declined from the first to the second, third and fourth term at university but there was still 18–30% incidence in the fourth year. There was no evidence of sex differences or age differences within the populations studied in the U.K. However, a recent study conducted in a boarding school situated in the mountains North-East of Melbourne in Australia (Fisher and Peacock, 1988) revealed an interesting result. The overall incidence for prompted report on a five category rating scale of frequency of homesickness experi-ence was 82% for females and 75% for males, but of those who reported frequent or very frequent feelings of homesickness 75% were female. The school places heavy emphasis on treking and outward bound activities, operates a seven-day working week and is isolated. It is possible that females are more affected by these conditions. (See later discussions in Chapter 8 on job strain in educational environments.)

THE SYNDROME OF HOMESICKNESS

The issue of whether homesickness is a sickness or disease is a difficult one. There is no evidence that it should be considered as a sickness because it appears to be a pattern of response to a specific life event. We have not explored the issue of whether there is an organic cause, but it seems likely that we are dealing with a pattern of mood and motivational change that is within the bounds of normal mechanisms.

This does not mean that we cannot identify a grouping of symptoms which characterise a syndrome. The correlations between self-reported elements concerned with grief for and yearning for home, family, and friends are high in the homesick (r_s 0.79; $p < 0.01$). Equally there are highly correlated symptoms such as obsessionality, anxiety, depression, somatic symptoms, and cognitive failure. The inter-correlations are not lower than 0.6 and all are significant. For this reason it would seem reasonable to regard homesickness as a form of post-traumatic stress syndrome following the transition from home.

SUMMARY AND CONCLUSIONS

In this chapter we have concentrated on some of the issues concerning the assessment and incidence of the homesickness syndrome. As was emphasised initially, we began working on a topic that had never been explored in any great depth. In the process we opened a Pandora's Box of problems, most of which had never been tackled in the literature on the measurements of other clinical states.

In general, the provision of a term for prompted questions markedly influences the reporting levels of homesickness; there is a step-function leap from under 20% to over 60% incidence. After that, however, format and styles of presentation, or mode of response did not further influence reporting. Homesickness is not socially sanctioned as an experience. It is not therefore acceptable in the way that the response to bereavement is. For this reason many people suffer without help. Lack of social acceptability may explain why the use of names on questionnaires reduces incidence level.

An unexpected finding was that, counter to initial expectations, there were no sex or age differences in homesickness reporting. The failure to find strong evidence of sex differences is particularly interesting in view of both the existing research literature and the results of our own studies which indicate the relative vulnerability of females to the stresses of university. However, a recent finding conducted in an Austrialian boarding school, situated in the mountains, has revealed a bias towards high frequency of the experience of homesickness in females. The issue is considered at greater length in Chapter 8 but it might be the case that the demanding physical activities of the school create too much strain for females and that the reporting of homesickness reflects this problem.

4 Episodic Homesickness Reporting: The Implications for Attentional Resources

There is an assumption underlying the measurement of mental disorder that the greater the level of the disorder the greater the number of different reported symptoms. This assumption is best described by an hierarchical model in which 'worse' implies an increasing range of qualitatively different signs. Although some questionnaires take note of intensity by the provision of a rating scale for each item, the assumption that intensity is expressed by range of symptoms as well is implicit.

In advance of the research, it was not possible to specify the symptoms and signs likely to be associated with homesickness. So the procedure followed was to rely on self-report assessment using simple category rating scales. A main aim was to collect data on all aspects of homesickness with a view to developing a validated questionnaire for assessment.

EPISODIC REPORTING CHARACTERISTICS

As already outlined in the previous chapter, diary formats were initially used for investigating homesickness in the first two weeks of a new term for university and boarding school students. The percentage returns were high for school pupils (100%) because although completions were anonymous, schools made arrangements to organise collections, but unacceptably low (20–30%) for university students. Thus most of what is to be outlined next is taken from the boarding school data.

It should be explained that there were problems in obtaining data on homesickness because it is often a problem for schools and is regarded as a 'sensitive' issue. Many school staff regarded homesickness as such a major difficulty at the beginning of the school year that there was an anxiety over whether reporting homesickness, however organised, would precipitate or encourage more widespread distress amongst pupils. A compromise was to use low subject numbers rather than sample a complete school cohort in case the fear of some schools that homesickness could be precipitated was justified. The technique of random sampling from lists of names was used to ensure that there was a minimal bias in the selected groups. All subjects provided written definitions of homesickness as described in the previous chapter.

Pilot studies on diary completion showed that when unsegmented columns were used, respondents tended to hatch-in specific zones against the time scale as representing periods during which they recalled feelings of homesickness. A proportion of about 5–15% filled in the complete column. In order to avoid problems due to poor indication of beginning and end of a hatched period on a column, therefore, the columns in the main diary studies were divided into hourly units and respondents were instructed to indicate by means of an 'X' in any one hour unit, whether or not homesickness had been experienced.

The results of the studies indicated that there were three types of reporting pattern. The first group did not make any entry at all in the homesickness column although in the appropriate diary format they listed problems and worry periods; therefore this was taken to be an indication of no homesickness rather than a failure to complete the diary.

The second group was labelled 'episodic reporters' in that some but not all of the cells were endorsed. About 60–70% of the sample was in this category. Reporting patterns were different for male as compared with female pupils in this group in that the former were more likely to report homesickness in the morning whereas the latter were more likely to report it in the evening. (The scale was restricted to 12 hours for school pupils as a concession to the school authorities.) Generally the data for the episodic homesickness groups suggest that the day's activities help to keep home-sick experiences at bay. This may be an important consideration for prevention or intervention; it does seem to be likely that keeping a pupil busy and enforcing commitment and interest may decrease the likelihood of continuous homesickness experience. The intermittency of the experi-ence may similarly be controllable in that the periods of experience may occur during passive moments, boring lessons, or undirected mental acitiv-ity. There is qualified support for the latter assertion. A diary format which required situational details surrounding the experience to be completed, indicated that mental (rather than physical) behaviour was vulnerable and that passivity (rather than activity) was associated (Fisher et al., 1986). However, passivity and engagement on mental tasks could be conse-quences as much as causes and there is no a priori way of checking this, because of the difficulty of working out exactly what a pupil should be doing for each hour of his or her school day.

The third group were non-episodic homesickness reporters in that the respondents endorsed every single cell of every day and on some occasions simply put an elongated 'X' right down all the cells of the column from top to bottom. It would appear that this group, accounting for about 10–15% of homesickness reporters, were continually homesick. They reported themselves as feeling very distressed.

THE COGNITIVE BASIS OF HOMESICKNESS EXPERIENCE

Microstructure of Fluctuating Psychological States

An aspect of distress and mental disorder which has not been analysed in any detail, is the change in qualitative and quantitative states over time. An assumption seems to be made that, for example, once depression occurs, whether acutely or chronically, there is a step-function change in psychological and biological factors. That is to say the main features of depression are presumed to be durable and stable in time unless there is therapy, intervention or the operation of unknown self limiting factors. However, descriptions of the (supposedly) non-clinical response to bereavement, emphasise the occurrence of adaption and changes in level and quality of periods of grief and emotionality (see Parkes, 1972). Perhaps we have not measured the daily changes in mood state in sufficient detail in clinical conditions.

The cognitive approach to the understanding of depression and anxiety assumes that mood states are precipitated and maintained by thought processes. Thus Beck (1967; 1970) describes the negative cognitive triad in which there is a bias towards pessimistic evaluations of the self and the future. Beck has also noted the way in which depressed or anxious states can be triggered by implanting the appropriate thoughts in the minds of patients and has indicated the prevalence of appropriately depressed or anxious thoughts in the dreams of patients. This might suggest that: (a) clinical states can be triggered from 'outside'—i.e. cues such as sounds and visual images or certain conversations can evoke mood states appropriate to the disorder; (b) clinical states can be maintained in the absence of relevant external cues because of the way the person views his world. Thus the depressed person creates a world of pessimistic and unhappy events. Eysenck (1988) has indicated that the anxious patient lives in a world of threats because of over-sensitivity to threat-related events.

One issue which is important is the implication for demands on the attentional resources. Theories of the effects of environmental stress on performance characteristics have emphasised the importance of the effects on attentional change because the external stressful event captures the attentional resource creating blocks or errors because of perceptual failure (see Broadbent, 1958; Fisher, 1986). Stresses such as life events may make comparable demands on attentional resource and may compete effectively with daily tasks for the domination of the resource (see Fisher, 1986).

Homesickness Frequency and Psychological Disturbance

From studies of diary reporting, it appears that in general both 'worrying' (Fisher, Frazer, & Murray, 1984; 1986) and 'experience of homesickness' occur in bouts or episodes. Unless it is very distressing, a problem would not necessarily worry a person for every moment of the day and night. Similarly, the majority of homesickness reporters tend to report discrete periods of concern, usually at the end or beginning of the day when these experiences occur. One possibility is that frequency of occurrence of a noted period of worry provides an index of the seriousness of the particular problem. Fisher, Frazer, and Murray (1984), and Fisher (1987) developed the idea of using worry levels and particularly the ratio of self-reported worries to problems for different problem categories as a means of examining level of distress created. On this analysis a problem is defined in terms of qualitative features of content and a worry unit represents a period of ruminative activity associated with the problem. The underlying rationale is that periods of rumination or worry created by a particular problem give an indication of how important and demanding that problem is. In the case of homesickness it would seem equally reasonable to suppose that *episodes of rumination* (or worry units) provide a useful measure of the magnitude of the effect. If this is the case, it might be easier to ask a subject how frequently he or she feels homesick than to ask how intense the experience of homesickness is.

There is of course no particular reason for arguing that homesickness is a special case of disorder—the above remarks could be extended to other disorders and fluctuating mood states. It is reasonable to suppose that depression and anxiety have episodic characteristics. The medical diagnosis merely bases decision as to clinical state on the range of symptoms and the intensity of the psychological and biological disruption involved. Measures such as frequency of episode are ignored. In considering and tackling the problem of assessing homesickness there is a Pandora's Box of issues which are of relevance to the process of clinical diagnosis.

One issue of interest is whether a frequency measure of homesickness relates to level of distress in terms of psychoneurotic symptoms. On the hypothesis that the self-reported frequency measure is a manifestation of level of disorder, then it should follow that we should find a high positive correlation. This could not be examined in the context of boarding school pupils because of the difficulties this might produce for the school authorities to parental consent. Also there was the problem of age; scales are designed to measure mental disorder in adults. However we were able to undertake a study involving first-year university students.

The study (to be published) involved 60 first-year residential students in the sixth week of the first term at the University of Dundee. All students who were approached took part in the study, and returned the questionnaires anonymously by post using the pre-stamped addressed envelopes supplied. Each respondent was asked to provide a written definition of homesickness and to indicate first whether or not he/she had experienced it. This provided the basis for a dichotic separation of subjects. Those who indicated that they had experienced homesickness, were then asked to indicate by means of a seven-point scale how frequently the experience had occurred from 'sometimes' through to 'all the time'. All subjects were asked to complete the Middlesex Hospital Questionnaire (designed by Crown & Crisp, 1966) which assesses psychoneurotic symptoms in the general population, and to complete the Cognitive Failure Questionnaire (designed by Broadbent, Cooper, Fitzgerald, & Parkes, 1982) which assesses absent-mindedness. The questionnaires were provided in random order to each participant.

Spearman's correlation statistics revealed that there were high positive correlations between self-reported frequency of homesickness and MHQ score overall ($r_s = 0.81$, $p < 0.001$) and with CFQ score ($r_s = 0.69$, $p < 0.001$). The MHQ subscores which correlated at greater than 0.5 with self-reported frequency of homesickness, were depression ($r_s = 0.62$, $p < 0.001$), anxiety ($r_s = 0.71$, $p < 0.001$), somatic symptoms ($r_s = 0.78$, $p < 0.001$), and obsessionality ($r_s = 0.89$, $p < 0.001$).

Table 4.1 further illustrates that separation into the two most extreme cells on the scale (one and two v. six and seven) produced scores on the MHQ and CFQ which were statistically significant in the direction of increased psychoneurotic symptom and cognitive failure level for the high as compared with low 'frequency of homesickness' (Mann Whitney 'U' Test significance level at least $p < 0.05$). Thus the frequency measure appears associated in the expected way with level of distress.

Taken collectively, these results support the hypothesis that *self-reported homesickness frequency* is positively associated with psychological distress and absent-mindedness. There are of course a number of possible explanations of why this should be the case; correlations do not imply causation, nor do they indicate the direction of causal processes (see Fisher, 1987). It

TABLE 4.1
Mental Distress and Absent-mindedness for Different Frequency
Levels of Homesickness Reporting (SD in Parentheses)

	Low Homesick Frequency Cells 1 & 2 (n = 18)	High Homesick Frequency Cells 6 & 7 (n = 10)
	$\bar{x}$	$\bar{x}$
Frequency	1.01 (0.10)	6.3 (0.16)
MHQ	25.9 (11.1)	31.6 (11.8)[a]
CFQ	39.8 (13.6)	45.6 (12.1)[a]

[a]$p < 0.01$.

remains possible that psychoneurotic disturbance and absent-mindedness create the preconditions for homesickness or that the symptoms are part of the homesickness reaction.

The high correlations of cognitive and distress symptoms suggest that we can refer to homesickness as a syndrome (although not necessarily an illness). The syndrome involves cognitive orientation to home in all aspects and distress symptoms such as depression, anxiety, phobic, and somatic complaints. These symptoms are also accompanied by high ruminative activity and perhaps partly in consequence, high absent-mindedness.

Homesickness and Attentional Resources

Ultimately we need to explain *the persistence of the ruminative content characteristic of homesickness in cognition*. The final explanation must involve the apparent domination of attention processes by such content. It appears as if a homesick person is 'living mentally' in a previous environment. This reflective state is not unlike the state of bereaved people who live with the memories of the deceased. Why does attention become dominated by the past in this way? We do not know whether the domination is unavoidable or avoidable. It is necessary to understand the principles of the capture of the mechanism.

The underlying assumption of most attentional models is that there is a fixed attentional resource, partly controlled by a person and partly subject to capture by external factors or unwanted thoughts. Threatening signals or emotional states are assumed to provide connotative signals which occupy the resource.

The capacity model of attention draws partly on the early work on mental load and partly on studies of dichotic listening and distraction (see Brown, 1964; Fisher, 1986, Chapter 7). It was assumed that processing resources, including attentional resources, are described by a fixed capacity system. Spare or reserve capacity is defined by the difference between capacity and the perceptual load imposed by a task. Reserve capacity cannot be indexed by single task performance because it will be within capacity and therefore error-free. However the addition of a secondary loading task will provide a means of assessing reserve capacity because, to the extent that the combined tasks exceed capacity, there will be errors.

Although dated and criticised because of the assumption that there is a non-expandable resource, nevertheless this approach provides the basis for a descriptive model of what appears to be true for the homesick. There is domination of a limited capacity attentional resource by thoughts of home and by the distress that results. An obvious question is why there is no domination of attention by the demands of the new life at school or university. One possibility is that the new environment simply fails to provide *effective competition*. This could be enhanced by behaviour; the homesick person is often withdrawn and uncommitted. It could also be created by an all pervasive distress state.

Hamilton (1974) pioneered an attempt to examine the effects of test anxiety in terms of the concept of spare capacity. Average processing capacity and spare processing capacity together define the available resource. It was assumed that stressful situations created by tests produce internal streams of signals which can compete for processing resources as effectively as external signals. As long as the available resource is greater than the requirement of those internal signals then performance is unaffected. Performance movement occurs when the resource is exceeded.

Figure 4.1 illustrates the possibility that there are competing streams of information requiring access to a limited capacity system. Compelling *external circumstances* may gain the attentional resource. Equally compelling *internal themes* may gain access to the resource. Just as we might expect a person to be unable to concentrate in the presence of high environmental demand (noise, glare, vibration etc.), we might also expect the person who has experienced a major life event to be preoccupied in that the attentional resource is captured by the processing of information about the particular threat. Perhaps periods of 'capture' of the attentional mechanism create the frequency characteristics of the disorder.

The Attentional Demands Model.   In order to understand the homesickness reporting patterns observed in the diaries of the boarding school pupils, two possible 'attentional resource' explanations are possible. The first, christened the 'demand-strength model' assumes that the non-homesick, episodic homesick, and non-episodic homesick differ quantitatively on a single dimension. As shown in the first part of Figure 4.1, it is assumed that competing home-directed information varies in strength and hence in its chances of capture of the attentional mechanism. For the non-homesick,

1. DEMAND STRENGTH MODEL

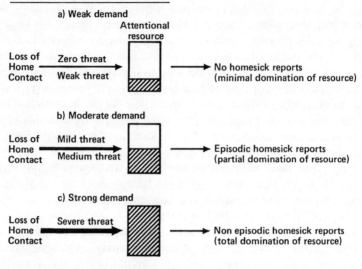

a) Weak demand

Attentional resource

Loss of Home Contact → Zero threat / Weak threat → No homesick reports (minimal domination of resource)

b) Moderate demand

Loss of Home Contact → Mild threat / Medium threat → Episodic homesick reports (partial domination of resource)

c) Strong demand

Loss of Home Contact → Severe threat → Non episodic homesick reports (total domination of resource)

2. COMPETING DEMANDS MODEL

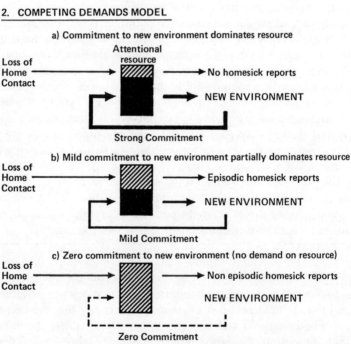

a) Commitment to new environment dominates resource

Attentional resource

Loss of Home Contact → → No homesick reports

NEW ENVIRONMENT

Strong Commitment

b) Mild commitment to new environment partially dominates resource

Loss of Home Contact → → Episodic homesick reports

NEW ENVIRONMENT

Mild Commitment

c) Zero commitment to new environment (no demand on resource)

Loss of Home Contact → → Non episodic homesick reports

NEW ENVIRONMENT

Zero Commitment

FIG. 4.1. Attentional demand models of homesickness reporting.

there is minimal interference from 'home' sources of information. For the episodic homesick reporters, homesick ruminative activity is assumed to be stronger and more demanding because of the effect of separation from home. For the non-episodic homesick, the dominance of the information is continuous because of the high level of threat created by the break with home.

There is evidence to support the idea that home thoughts provide an intrusive source of worry material for pupils newly residential at a new school. A diary study concerned only with recording problems (Fisher, Frazer, & Murray, 1984) showed that although the proportion of school-orientated worries ('will teacher like me'; 'coping with maths lessons'; 'finding my kilt jacket for church'; 'being bullied') was greater than home-orientated worries ('is the dog OK?'; 'hope my mother is alright without me'; 'who is feeding the fish?' 'my brother's illness'), school orientated problem/worry ratios were significantly greater than the home-orientated problem/worry ratios. This is illustrated in Table 4.2 which shows the problem/worry ratio based on the number of worries to problems. This suggests that home does have a profound effect on the thoughts of pupils although they are living in a new environment and may be part of the normal adaptation to a move away from home. This will be discussed again in a later context, but as far as the attentional demand model outlined above is concerned, the data are supportive of the idea that home-based thoughts are likely to have the capacity to dominate attention. All that needs to be assumed is that the level of ruminative activity reflects the level of threat created by the break with home.

The Competing Demands Model.   By contrast, an alternative concep-tualisation is the competing demands model illustrated in Fig. 4.1. This assumes that *the new environment* is the critical factor because it has the

TABLE 4.2
Frequencies of School-orientated and Home-orientated Problems and Associated Worry Units (in Parentheses); $N = 50$

	School-orientated	Home-orientated	Unclassified	Total
Frequency	304 (641)	75 (233)	9 (12)	388 (886)
$\bar{x}$	6.1 (12.8)	1.5 (4.7)	—	7.8 (17.72)
SD	7.3	3.6	—	8.9
Percentage	78.4	19.3	2.3	100.0
P/W ratio	0.58	0.26	—	0.56

Ratio of number worry units per reported problem calculated for each individual subject.

potential to create an information source which swamps the attentional resource, thus keeping homesick thoughts attenuated. Exposure to the novel environment following a transition provides a need for learning new faces, locations, routines. The demands of the new environment thus could swamp the attentional resource leaving little capacity available for homesick thoughts. The model will give a plausible account of why episodic homesickness reporters are more likely to report homesickness on awakening or at night, because the day's activities at school create the competing sources of information. Equally, the finding of an association of homesickness with passivity is understandable in that the act of being passive may mean that there is less demand and therefore less competition for the attentional resource. The finding in the same study that homesickness is more likely during 'mental' as compared with 'physical' tasks could be interpreted in much the same way. Mental tasks may require acts of concentration to maintain demand. Early work by Bills (1931) established basic data on blocks in a colour-naming task and showed that task monotony is a major factor in determining the frequency of block occurrence.

The competing demands model assumes that homesick and non-homesick groups *differ in terms of their ability to become committed*. Fisher (1985; 1986) argued that demand is not a passive property of situations but is an interactional concept which depends on engaging the task. An academic examination is not threatening if a person has no aim to pass it. Although in some highly structured and controlled environments such as military training establishments and some robust public schools, activity is imposed, in many cases particularly with university and college life the student must *self-create* demands. If a student fails to attend lectures or tutorials the system may not necessarily operate immediate sanctions. Commitment is therefore, to a great extent, self-determined.

Klinger (1975) denotes 'current concern' as a state of sensitivity to a particular problem or task. Commitment is the onset of current concern. Consummation or disengagement terminates the concern. In terms of this descriptive analysis, the homesick may be those who fail to have a current concern which is university- or school-related. The competing demands model provides a means of distinguishing the three groups (non-homesick; episodic homesick; non-episodic homesick) in a way which implies qualitative distinctions based on level of commitment following tansition. All three groups are assumed to be subjected *to the same level of disruption produced by the separation from home and loss of contact with loved family and friends or routines*, but the non-homesick *create activity which attenuates the dominance of resulting ruminative activity*. The episodic homesick are partially able to do this making use of the demands of the day's activities. By comparison the non-episodic homesick are unable to do this and as a result they are mentally swamped by unremitting homesick ruminations. This fits with the phenomenological descriptions obtained from non-episodic homesick reporters: 'I cannot stop thinking about home'; 'It seems strange, but I am mentally living my life at home'; 'All day my thoughts centre on what I would be doing if I were at home. It fills me with pain and distress'; 'I cannot even start to get involved here. I just think of home'.

Thus a picture which might be valid is one in which there is some effect of separation and loss for most people but the challenge of new opportunities creates commitments which help to keep any unhappiness at bay. Those who are not disposed to take on the challenge are handicapped in terms of the potential for attenuating the effects of separation and loss. This notion will be considered again in later chapters.

SUMMARY AND CONCLUSIONS

The syndrome of homesickness is associated with cognitions centred on the event of leaving home, family and friends. The degree to which cognition is dominated by the previous environment is variable. For some, the domination appears from self-report in diaries to be total. These people we have referred to as 'non-episodic reporters' because they appear not to experience episodes but to be swamped by the experience. Distress levels appear to relate closely to the degree to which cognition is dominated by home thoughts.

A descriptive formulation perhaps provides a framework for understanding the effect. If we imagine a limited capacity attentional resource, then we can account for the differences in the level of experience by assuming that *the break with home varies in its capacity to threaten a person.* This 'demand-strength' model (see Fig. 4.1) assumes that the demands or threats created by situations differentially swamp resources (or are differentially resisted by resources).

However, the 'competing demands' model assumes that the demand or threat does not differentiate individuals; leaving home is stressful for all. What makes the difference is *the degree to which a person can become committed to the new environment.* High levels of commitment mean that attention is externally dominated and homesick thoughts are kept at bay. Since the day's activities play a part in this, then it would be reasonable to expect bimodal distributions of homesickness reporting where, for mildly homesick people, periods of inactivity allow homesick thoughts to temporarily dominate the resource.

By contrast the severely homesick would be expected to have low commitment to the new environment so that homesickness continues to dominate.

This is in addition to the possibility of a positive feedback loop: homesickness → lack of commitment → homesickness. The intriguing question is therefore whether the state of homesickness worsens or whether there are identifiable events which break the cycle. Vulnerable individuals would be those least able to enter into commitments rapidly following transition.

5

The Correlates of Homesickness: Associated Psychological States and Health

In this chapter, we explore in greater detail the correlates of the syndrome of homesickness. In the previous chapter it was established that there appear to be a number of highly correlated cognitive and distress symptoms in those who self-report homesickness. A possibility already considered is that as in the grief reaction, the specific environmental event drives the cognitive state which is characterised by preoccupation with the home environment. This may be a specific manifestation of post-traumatic stress syndrome. There is none of the bitter-sweet experience of nostalgia; instead it appears that the preoccupations serve to drive intense feelings of unhappiness accompanied by anxiety and depression. Absent-mindedness would be expected to increase as a function of accompanying ruminative activity.

In this chapter there is some further exploration of the nature of the syndrome. An hierarchical model is envisaged in which a possible scheme of events is: (a) transition; (b) the focus of cognitive activity on home; (c) the symptoms of distress, disturbance and absent-mindedness. However, another event could drive similar distress and absent-mindedness. The distinguishing factors concern cognitive orientations. There is some support for this view since it is the cognitive symptoms (missing, preoccupation with home, yearning for home) that distinguishes the homesick from the non-homesick group on the Dundee Relocation Inventory ('DRI'), a scale designed by Fisher and Murray (in press, see footnote, p. 123) to measure homesickness.

HOMESICKNESS, PSYCHOLOGICAL DISTURBANCE, AND HEALTH

Studies of university students reporting homesickness (Fisher et al., 1985; Fisher & Hood, 1987) have indicated that they are distinguished from their non-homesick counterparts by raised levels of psychoneurotic scores on non-clinical scales such as the Middlesex Hospital Questionnaire ('MHQ'; Crown & Crisp, 1966) and raised absent-mindedness scores on the Cognitive Failure Questionnaire ('CFC'; Broadbent et al., 1982). Taken collectively, the practical implication is that the homesick person is distressed and likely to behave non-effectively in the new environment. Perhaps not surprisingly, the evidence from both the above studies also indicates poorer adaptation to university life as assessed by the College Adaptation Questionnaire ('CAQ'; Crombag, 1968).

Because the topic of homesickness has been largely unresearched, it is useful at this stage to consider the main features of the syndrome in some detail. We have chosen to present the data where appropriate because there may be readers who wish to research the topic further. Readers who want only general impressions of main findings could disregard the tabulated material and read only the general statements in the text.

There are three main sets of correlates to consider as part of the syndrome:

1. Accompanying psychoneurotic symptoms (these might be cause or consequence of the cognitive response to an environmental event).
2. Absent-mindedness; there are several explanations of increased absent-mindedness in stress.
3. Physical health changes; there are several explanations of how health changes might link to psychological state.

Psychoneurotic Symptoms

The Middlesex Hospital Questionnaire was used for the assessment of psychological state because it is a short diagnostic test for non-clinical populations and because it does not prejudge the types of symptoms which will occur in a particular condition. A range of short subscales, include depression, anxiety, phobias, hysteria, obsessionality and somatic symptoms.

As illustrated by Table 5.1, a longitudinal study by Fisher and Hood (1987) showed that, following the transition to university, the symptoms which are elevated in the homesick are depression, obsessional symptoms, somatic symptoms, and anxiety. Overall, the level of psychoneurotic symptoms (MHQ) is raised following transition.

TABLE 5.1
Cognitive Failure, Mental Health, and Adjustment Profiles Before and
After the Transition in Homesick and Non-homesick Residents[a]

	Not Homesick (n = 42)		Homesick (n = 22)	
	$\bar{\chi}$	SD	$\bar{\chi}$	SD
At Home				
MHQ1	22.81	(8.6)	29.2^c	(12.5)
Obsessional (personality)	2.61	(2.2)	3.72^b	(2.7)
Somatic	3.21	(2.5)	4.54^b	(2.7)
Depression	1.89	(1.6)	3.82^c	(2.8)
CFQ1	32.64	(10.66)	36.9NS	(12.3)
Sixth Week at University				
MHQ2	23.0	(11.54)	33.04^c	(14.1)
Anxiety	3.78	(3.1)	6.48^c	(3.7)
Somatic	2.63	(2.1)	5.17^d	(2.9)
Depression	2.56	(2.3)	4.48^c	(3.2)
Obsessional (symptoms)	2.54	(1.6)	3.35^b	(2.1)
CFQ2	38.21	(11.88)	42.78NS	(13.5)
CAQ	100.69	(17.7)	84.31^d	(18.2)
DRI	4.0	(3.2)	8.50^d	(4.2)

[a]As designed by 'not homesick' versus three other categories of 'homesick' on self-rating scale (from Fisher & Hood, 1987).
[b]$p < 0.05$.
[c]$p < 0.01$.
[d]$p < 0.001$.

Figure 5.1 illustrates a comparable finding, reported by Fisher and Frazer (1988), for student nurses. A longitudinal study was conducted in which student nurses were assessed prior to leaving home, after six weeks in nursing college, and during first (medical) and second (surgical) ward experience. As Fig. 5.1 shows, the effect of the transition to nursing college was to produce an increase in psychological disturbance and absent-mindedness. The effect was greater than any effect of ward experience although obsessionality increased on the surgical ward. The flattening off of scores at the time of ward experience did not appear to be a ceiling effect. The symptom increases shown by the nurses were similar to those shown by the students; in particular, there were increases in obsessionality and depression.

In a study of homesickness in 357 first year students at Manchester University, Kane (1987) reported homesickness incidence levels of 50% initially (on arrival) and 37% in the fourth week of term. As shown in

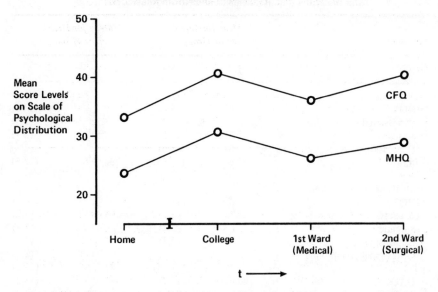

FIG. 5.1   The stress of the transition to nursing college (Fisher & Frazer, 1988).

Table 5.2, homesick individuals were found to have greater disturbance scores on the General Health Questionnaire ('GHQ') and specifically greater scores on somatic symptoms, anxiety, social dysfunction and depression. Kane also reported that, as rated on three-category rating scales, the homesick were less satisfied with friends and social life ($p < 0.01$) and

TABLE 5.2
Manchester Study on General Health in Homesick and Non-homesick
Students (from Kane, 1987)

	Non-homesick Mean Score	Homesick Mean Score
GHQ	2.91	5.20[a]
Somatic symptoms	1.23	1.85[a]
Anxiety	0.72	1.35[a]
Social dysfunction	0.77	1.61[a]
Depression	0.18	0.39[b]
Short inventory of minor lapses	2.09	2.23[a]

[a]$p < 0.01$.
[b]$p < 0.05$.

TABLE 5.3
The Manchester Study on High- and Low-error Groups and Associated
Psychological Health Variables (from Kane, 1987)

Variables	Mean for Low-error Group	Mean for High-error Group
GHQ	2.78	4.69[a]
Somatic symptoms	1.71	1.73[a]
Anxiety	0.67	0.23[a]
Social dysfunction	0.74	1.41[a]
Depression	0.16	0.38[a]
Homesick	0.33	0.49[b]

[a] $p < 0.01$.
[b] $p < 0.05$.

less satisfied with academic life ($p < 0.01$). Finally, as shown in Table 5.2 they had higher scores on Short Inventory of Minor Lapses developed by Reason and Lucas, 1982.

Kane also divided the subjects into high-error reporters (greater than the mean) on the Short Inventory of Minor Lapses and low-error reporters (equal to or less than the mean). As shown in Table 5.3, *the high-error reporters* had high scores on GHQ, and on the somatic, anxiety, social dysfunction and depression subscores, as well as for homesickness. Taken collectively, the studies of both Fisher and Hood (1987) and Kane (1987) establish that homesickness may reduce the likelihood of efficient coping with and adapting to the demands of university life.

The Fisher and Hood study provided an unexpected result: When the data obtained from the students two months prior to leaving home for university were examined, it was found that the homesick and non-homesick groups differed in that *overall psychoneurotic scores and specifically depression, somatic and obsessionality scores were already elevated in the potentially homesick.* This might suggest the existence of a personal or circumstantial vulnerability factor. Covariate analysis established that *anxiety* and *obsessionality symptoms* interacted with the transition.

The differentiation of homesick and non-homesick prior to transition might be early signs of vulnerability in the homesick. However, the factors which indicate vulnerability are not the factors which interact with the transition: depression distinguishes the two groups but does not interact with the move; anxiety does not distinguish the groups initially (at home) but does interact with the move.

There are a number of possible explanations of apparent vulnerability factors. The first is that the potentially homesick person fears the transition ahead and begins to manifest signs of distress in advance. The human capacity for anticipating and manifesting distress and incompetence on current tasks due to a percieved impending threat, is well documented (see Wherry & Curran, 1965; Fisher, 1984).

The second possibility is that the potentially homesick person is more distressed whilst still at home, because of a previous experience. Most university students have probably been through a difficult and demanding school year, frequently involving crucial summer examinations (although for Scottish students this is less likely because the last year at school involves sixth year studies and is devoid of critical examinations). Even if a student already has artificially elevated scores, this is not against the vulnerability hypothesis. In other words, vulnerability may result from a previous treatment of stress which creates a psychological state not conducive to coping with further pressures.

The nature of vulnerability and its relationship with ill health is little understood. Brown reports that early parental loss may create a change in the level of care a child receives and may influence, via intermediate behaviours, the risk of adverse response such as depression in relation to a stress later in life (see Brown, 1988). The difference in this case is really only the *temporal distance* between the predisposing factor (early parental loss) and the response to a later precipitant. In the case of the person vulnerable to homesickness following the transition to university, the predisposing factors might be more immediate (recent examination stress at school). Cumulative 'precipitant-precipitant' effects are implicitly proposed in the Holmes and Rahe (1965) *Schedule of Recent Experiences*, designed to provide an arithmetic weighting of life events which predict the risk of illness in terms of an additive model (e.g. see Rahe, 1988).

Finally, the raised level of psychoneurotic scores prior to leaving home, may be a manifestation of emotionality/insecurity which renders a person vulnerable to transitions of various kinds. In particular, depression appears to be predictive of homesickness after the transition, but does not itself interact with the move. A possible explanation considered later in the book is that the depressed are vulnerable because of their disposition to remain uncommitted to the move and the new environment.

The finding that there may be ways of predicting homesickness in advance is of obvious importance for the targeting of limited resources on newly residential students. Pre-transition depression might be the key predictor in this respect.

Absent-mindedness

Studies by Fisher et al. (1985) and by Fisher and Hood (1987) showed that cognitive failure levels were significantly raised in those who reported homesickness. Moreover, Fisher and Hood (1987) reported raised cognitive failure scores in all students, following the transition to university (in the context of the longitudinal study referred to in the previous section). However, the difference in absent-mindedness scores was not significant for the homesick group. Collectively, the results support the hypothesis that the transition to university is a stressful experience which creates increased absent-mindedness, and that in general the level of absent-mindedness is likely to be greater in the homesick students. Reports from homesick university students (Fisher et al., 1985) indicate that about one-third of the group experienced loss of concentration, had poor attendance at lectures, or handed in work late.

There were also significant positive correlations between the *frequency* measure of homesickness (how frequently homesickness episodes are experienced, as reported on a five-category rating scale) and the degree to which work was reported as affected (0.46); the degree to which there was lack of concentration (0.47); work handed in late (0.42). (All correlations significant at at least $p < 0.05$.)

The explanation of the effect of the transition on level of absent-mindedness is difficult. Since *all* students show a rise in score level following the transition relative to levels at home (Fisher & Hood, 1987) any explanation must take account of this. One possibility is that the transition to university is stressful for all students who undertake it, irrespective of whether they leave home or remain home-based, and that absent-mindedness reflects the increased stress. The second possibility is that leaving home *creates a step-function change in demand*—new faces and locations have to be learned, new procedures and rules have to be mastered because university environments are very different from school environments. Analysis of problems reported by students has indicated that difficulties associated with academic pressures, organisational factors and financial problems are paramount. Maybe cognitive efficiency levels do not change but demand on cognitive systems increases.

A laboratory-based study however, suggested that efficiency levels in performance might be altered in the homesick. A group of university students reporting homesickness but with scores of less than eight on the Beck Depression Inventory ($\bar{x} = 7.1$; SD $= 2.1$) was compared with a group of depressed (but not homesick) students scoring more than eight ($\bar{x} = 15.9$; SD $= 3.6$) and also with non-homesick, non-depressed controls ($\bar{x} = 3.9$; SD $= 3.1$). The study enabled partitioning into *actual performance, perceived performance* and *overall estimates of performance*. Subjects were required to type an overlearned word 'INITIATION' on the keyboard of a computer and, in the absence of visual feedback, to decide whether the word had been typed perfectly correctly or not. Subjects were required to indicate this by means of a bi-modal decision 'YES' or 'NO'. This procedure was repeated for 100 word trials. Then at the end of the

TABLE 5.4
Error Production and Detection in the Homesick and the Depressed

	Non-homesick (n = 14)		Homesick (n = 14)		Depressed (n = 14)	
	$\bar{\chi}$	SD	$\bar{\chi}$	SD	$\bar{\chi}$	SD
Typing errors produced	7.1	(3.1) ($p < 0.05$)	12.9	(2.9) (NS)	9.2	(2.6)
Errors in detection	5.3	(1.8) ($p < 0.01$)	13.1	(3.2) ($p < 0.05$)	6.0	(2.9)
Errors estimated (out of 100)	8.4	(0.9) ($p < 0.001$)	29.6	(7.8) (NS)	30.9	(6.8)

NOTE: p values represent the results of comparison of groups on Mann Whitney 'U' Tests.

task, subjects were required to assess overall how many errors they had made out of the 100 trials (overall assessment).

As Table 5.4 shows, the homesick subjects made more errors than the control group and made more wrong reports in this respect. This proved to be significant on a Kruskall Wallis, One-way Analysis of Variance ($0.05 > p > 0.01$). In common with the depressed group, and compared to the control group they over-estimated their overall error reports relative to errors actually reported trial by trial. These results suggest that there are different performance-related cognitions in the homesick. They appear close as a group to the depressed and, as MHQ scores suggest, they do generally portray high levels of depressive symptoms.

One possibility is that homesick subjects are more error prone because the intrusion of thoughts of home creates demands which interfere with the processing of information from other tasks. Homesick ruminations may render a person liable to inefficiency in daily life because of the reduction of attentional resources available. This fits with the picture of the homesick person as someone likely to be vague, error prone and generally not geared to cope with demands of university life. In turn this may create a positive feedback loop whereby the individual becomes inefficient and, far from becoming committed and involved in the new environment, experiences high demand and low control as a result. In turn this would mean that the chances are low of the new environment providing suitable information which can encourage commitment and which competes successfully with intrusive homesick thoughts. Thus, there is the possibility of a knock-on effect potentially leading to a point of personal crisis unless by circumstance or intervention the situation is changed. Again, resources need to be targeted effectively on students in such a way as to prevent this from happening. Screening for adverse response by student interviews with counsellors may well save resources later in the year.

Physical Health

As reported above, there are signs that homesickness is associated with ill health. There are elevated somatic symptoms on both the Middlesex Hospital Questionnaire and the General Health Questionnaire (Fisher & Hood, 1987; Kane, 1987). The latter research indicates an association with somatic symptoms. Table 5.5 shows the results of a study conducted retrospectively, at the end of the first school year on 117 boarding school pupils (all female, ages 11–14 years). The results indicate that there were more days off school for non-traumatic illness for the homesick group as compared with the non-homesick group. Equally, the homesick group had seen a doctor more times. There was no similar difference for the reporting of traumatic ailments such as sprains, breakages, contusions, cuts, and grazes. This latter finding argues against an explanation in terms of reporting bias.

A similar finding (Fisher & Peacock, 1988) occurred in the context of an Australian boarding school, famous for its emphasis on outward bound activity. Those reporting frequent or very frequent levels of homesickness reported a greater number of non-traumatic ailments. There was no difference in the reporting of traumatic ailments.

TABLE 5.5
Variables Associated with Homesickness Reports for Boarding School
Pupils (from Fisher et al., 1986)

Variable	Homesick (n = 83)		Non-homesick (n = 34)	
	$\bar{\chi}$	SD	$\bar{\chi}$	SD
Non-traumatic ailments	2.95	1.62	2.38[a]	1.28
Days affected	27.28	45.72	14.53[a]	12.71
Activities affected	3.94	11.59	6.09(NS)	10.16
Number of times doctor seen	1.88	1.49	1.32[a]	1.17
Traumatic ailments	0.06	0.24	0.09(NS)	0.29
Days affected	1.95	10.99	1.53(NS)	5.23
Activities affected	1.95	11.11	0.73(NS)	3.68
Number of times doctor seen	0.06	0.24	0.09(NS)	0.29

[a]$p < 0.05$.
Note: Larger means indicated higher scores on the attributes listed.
NS = not significant.

Explanation of the association is difficult. Perhaps when ill, a person is more likely to be homesick. This would fit in with the attentional model suggested in the previous chapter, since the person is withdrawn from daily activities which might suppress the homesick thoughts. Moreover, the need for love and comfort may be greater when an individual is unwell and therefore the 'missing' of parental contact is greater. Against this explanation is the finding that there are no comparable differences for traumatic ailments—because the above arguments apply equally to a child immobilised with a broken ankle. However, the table also shows that there are less reported traumatic, compared with non-traumatic, ailments per person. This is significant statistically and may be a factor which is influential.

An alternative explanation and one which fits with the recent research literature on life events and health (see Fisher, 1988) is that homesickness is a distressing experience and creates increased risk of ill health. Apparent ill health may be a direct consequence of pathological levels of arousal due to stressful experience. For example, high arousal might create headaches due to the change in the pattern of blood flow to the head, dizziness and nausea due to the over stimulation of the vagus nerve etc. In other words there might be arousal-linked symptoms which impair well-being.

Epidemiological evidence has already established that a number of psychosocial factors influence the risk of ill health. For example, marital status is a factor in illness. As shown in Fig. 5.2, the single and divorced are more at risk for various forms of ill health and aberrant behaviours as compared with the married (data replotted from Berkson, 1962). This finding alone indicates the possible importance of psychosocial mediators in the risk of illness, although the causal relationships are not clear.

A number of models have been proposed to account for the possible relationship between stressful experience and ill health. Totman (1979) argues that a transition or change can create a breakdown of role expectancies which is stressful to the individual. Dodge and Martin (1970) also favour an hypothesis based on the breakdown of social rules and emphasise the importance of status inconsistency as a factor creating stress.

Fisher (1986) presented a 'control model' of the relationship between stress and illness. It was argued from experimental evidence provided by Frankenhaeuser and Johansson (1982) that levels of cortisol (the distress hormone) are more likely to be high if a demanding task is characterised by low control. Thus, high demand and high control will be associated with raised effort, low distress, and high catecholamines; high demand and low control will be associated with raised effort and distress and high catecholamines and cortisol.

The presence of high levels of cortisol and adrenocorticotropic hormome (ACTH) responsible for its secretion, have been shown to increase the risk of suppression of the immune response and hence the risk of infectious

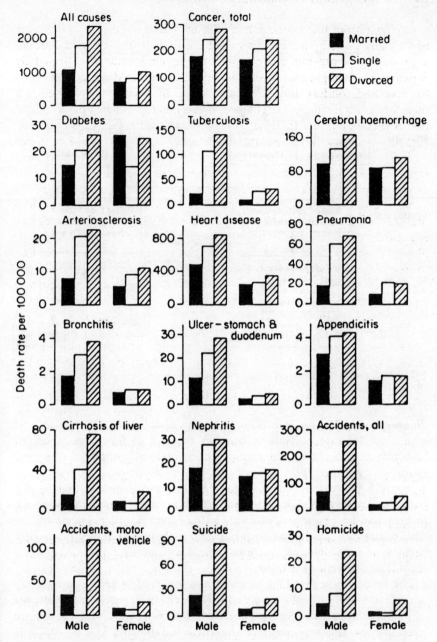

FIG. 5.2. Marital status and health—standardised death rates for different causes of death in the United States. Data redrawn from Berkson, 1962, with the permission of the American Medical Association (Fisher, 1986).

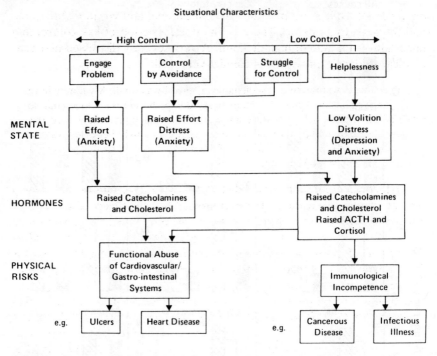

FIG. 5.3.   Conceptualisation of demand control relationships, hormone levels, and health (Fisher, 1986).

illness or opportunistic infections becoming established. The presence of high levels of catecholamines increases the risk of functional abuse of bodily systems such as the cardiovascular system leading to structural changes (see Fisher, 1986).

Figure 5.3 illustrates the possibility that for a high demand situation, the perception of level of control influences both mental state and the hormone balance and hence the risk of short- or long-term disorder. Fisher argued that conditions which favour prolonged pathological states of arousal because of high demand and low control will increase the risk of both chronic and infectious disease.

The formulation that high demand and low control create distress,fits with the model of job strain proposed by Karasek (1979) based on assessments of job environments by Swedish and American workers. Job strain is more likely in environments where demand is high and control is low. By contrast, high demand accompanied by high control is more likely to be accompanied by the experience of challenge and positive feelings.

One possibility is that homesickness creates protracted experience of distress in some individuals because of the conflict between the need to stay on at school, college or university for educational and vocational reasons, and the need to go home. There is, in effect, a period of low control and uncertainty at a time of high demand. A very severely distressed first-year medical student expressed this conflict very well:

> I have always wanted to do medicine ever since I was small. My family have always been in medicine. So I am here, doing the course I love, but so desperately homesick because I am 380 miles from home and I hate this place. I cannot find the things I like to do. I cry every night because I want to go home and I only stay on because of the medical course. I would never get in anywhere else now. It is all too late.

Conflict can create a protracted stressful experience and thus there is a further advantage for the increased risk of ill health. The person is locked into a situation possibly of his or her own making, in which the severance of direct contact with home although reversible, is *in effect perceived as irreversible*, because of the costs attached to reversing it. The result is distress which is prolonged, intense and likely to be frequent and continuous. Biological states would be expected to reflect this.

A further precondition for infectious disorder is contact with antigens. One aspect of the behaviour of the homesick which might *reduce* the risk of antigen contact is the tendency to withdraw and not take on commitments. This may explain the difference between the school and university populations in terms of self-reported ill health. The school pupil is less able to withdraw socially. He or she is more likely to be sharing a dormitory and is in any case generally involved in structured routines. The student is more able to stay in his or her room and to appear only for lectures or tutorials, although since the first university classes tend to be large, even lecture attendance may be avoided. There is a case for arguing that for equal levels of 'immuno-incompetence' brought about by raised stress hormone levels, the school and university populations may have different risks associated with antigen encounter because of life style differences.

SEX DIFFERENCES IN PSYCHOLOGICAL DISTURBANCE

With the exception of homesickness reports in an Australian boarding school (Fisher & Peacock, 1988), homesickness reporting does not generally differentiate the sexes. However as illustrated in Table 5.6, studies have revealed sex differences in both level of psychoneurotic symptoms and level of cognitive failure; females have raised scores on both sets of measures (Fisher & Hood, 1988; Hood, MacLachlan, & Fisher, 1987).

There is substantial research literature in the area of mental disorder which has established that there are sex differences in incidence and

TABLE 5.6
Sex Differences in Psychoneurotic Scores and Absent-mindedness in
First Year Students Following the Transition to University. From Hood,
MacLachlan, and Fisher (1987)

	Males (n = 189)		Females (n = 153)	
	$\bar{\chi}$	SD	$\bar{\chi}$	SD
MHQ total	24.1	(10.5)	29.2	(10.9)[b]
Anxiety	3.9	(3.1)	5.9	(3.5)[b]
Obsessional (persons)	2.9	(2.3)	3.1	(2.3)NS
Obsessional (symptoms)	2.6	(1.7)	2.7	(1.6)NS
Somatic	3.2	(2.5)	3.6	(2.5)NS
Depression	6.1	(3.2)	6.1	(3.4)NS
Phobia	2.7	(2.1)	4.3	(2.7)[b]
Hysteria	2.7	(2.5)	3.5	(2.5)[b]
CFQ	38.9	(12.7)	42.3	(13.3)[a]

[a] $p < 0.05$.
[b] $p < 0.001$.
NOTE: All probabilities are two-tailed.

magnitude of effect. Department of Health and Social Security figures indicate that about 40% more females than males are psychiatric cases, although there are diagnostic differences. More females than males are likely to be depressed, or to be treated for psychoneurotic symptoms. The difference is greater than 100% (e.g. see details provided by Cochrane, 1983).

Explanations of such well-established differences are varied. The suggestion that there are biological reasons would indicate that there should be more consistency in different social groups and over time, than is apparent. Moreover, mood changes which may be associated with, for example post-natal states or pre-menstrual tension, could not account for a large effect on random sampling. There are also sex and marital status interactions in that, as noted by Cochrane, in terms of mental disorder females are less protected by marital status than males. This again makes it difficult to assume that there is a basic vulnerability factor which is biologically based.

The possibility remains that the sex role has a direct influence on mood state. In traditional roles, the dominant male has more power and mastery than the female and this may mean that females are more readily helpless in society. If females depend for their rewards on being able to please other people, this is unpredictable and therefore is a low control experience. Against this is the data which suggest that the increased female propensity to mental disorder is a relatively recent phenomenon. It would be expected that since overall, women's roles have changed substantially in the direction of equality in the last 30 years, if anything their control over the environment should have increased. To counter this, it might be argued that the recent emergence of women into potentially important positions in western culture creates direct competition in which women fare less well in general; thus the contrasts may be exacerbated for all but the successful few.

Explanations in terms of self-esteem (not unlinked to the sex role issue) also need investigation. Low self-esteem individuals are less likely to cope with stressful life events, more likely to encounter stresses and are more difficult to help in terms of coping strategies (see Howarth & Dussuyer, 1988). Thus it is possible that females are more vulnerable in competitive environments because of the self-esteem factor. We would then expect increased possibility of helplessness.

Inter-personal skills may be limited in that the female sex role has traditionally encouraged being pleasant and rewarding. Yet confrontation over critical issues may be an important part of the progression in hierarchical work environments. Those who are tough and not easily swayed by adverse opinion may be rewarded. Therefore, the sex role may again render females relatively helpless with regard to the achievement of personal goals.

One interesting set of contradictions from the work on homesickness is that females: (1) do not generally report more homesickness; (2) report more signs of psychoneurotic disorder; (3) adapt better to university (on the College Adaptation Questionnaire designed by Crombag, 1968). Taken collectively, these results suggest the females to be stressed at the new challenges they face but reacting positively. The source of their increased distress may be the challenge, the extra effort required and the fear of failure rather than the loss of contact with home.

A less comprehensive explanation is that homesick females express emotional symptoms more readily than homesick males, and that the distress levels are consequently higher. However, we found no evidence of the interaction of sex and homesickness factors in psychoneurotic symptoms.

Overall, the results do suggest that females are more stressed by the transition to university. They even report moves as more stressful than their male counterparts. Yet the reasons for the stress might be different with a heavier 'job strain' element and they do show greater adaptation to university. As indicated earlier in this book the one finding of increased homesickness in females in the Australian boarding school may have been due to the high demand for strenuous treking and physical activity which may have proved less acceptable for females.

An interesting additional point is that raised level of psychoneurotic symptoms is *not a necessary condition for a homesick response*. As argued above, raised stress may be associated with the struggle for control and females more than males may respond with anxiety to the challenge of university. The competing demands model is given some support by this since increased commitment for females would result in competing information which helps to attenuate homesickness. The superior adaptation of females (College Adaptation Questionnaire) may reflect such increased commitment.

THEORETICAL SPECULATIONS

In this chapter we have pursued in some detail the symptoms associated with the homesickness syndrome. It is clear that there is raised psychological disturbance in the homesick and it maybe that this is cause or consequence of the cognitive state which is created by the act of leaving home. An obvious conclusion is that the distress is created by preoccupation with home and simultaneous realisation that home is now a long way away. The increased psychoneurotic symptoms, absent-mindedness and ill health might all be considered to be symptoms resulting from the domination of the themes in cognition. Perhaps mental health is organised on an hierarchical basis in which the main features of the cognitive state drive common symptoms in which idiosyncracies feature. Thus failure-cognitions will be distinguished from loss-cognitions; the theme of cognition contains the flavour of the event (failure or loss).

Unexpectedly, the longitudinal study began to provide some new clues; both home-based and residential students showed raised depression, obsessionality and absent-mindedness, suggesting that even for those not leaving home, the transition to university is very stressful. This began to provide the hint that the envrionment might have an important role to play in the reaction pattern of a new student. This is developed further in later chapters.

An obvious question to try to answer, having scrutinised research findings on the syndrome of homesickness, is whether the reaction pattern provides clues as to overall cause. It was made clear when different theories of the stressful effects of transition were described in Chapter 2, that it would be difficult to establish changes in the dependent variable which would enable us to identify a particular explanation.

However, there are some clues worth emphasising. The control theory could be argued to make different predictions than theories based on separation and loss, interruption, and role change. Control theory predicts *raised helplessness and depression* following a transition because of transient loss of control. In fact *all* students in the Fisher and Hood study, whether resident or not and whether homesick or not showed a substantial rise in depression, obsessional symptoms and absent-mindedness. This was also true for the student nurses studied by Fisher and Frazer (1988).

Perhaps the experience of transient loss of control is very much a feature of transitions for all who experience them. Obsessionality could be a manifestation of perceived helplessness or the overwhelming effect of the demands of the new environment. Absent-mindedness would be expected to reflect obsessionality.

However, the longitudinal study by Fisher and Hood seemed against the control hypothesis in that it was *anxiety* that interacted with the transition for the homesick residents. Raised anxiety is predicted by loss, interruption and role theories. This gives some support to the idea that the break with home is influential. A multi-causal or composite model is needed which focuses *both* on the impact of loss of direct contact with home and the transient loss of control in a high demand environment.

SUMMARY AND CONCLUSIONS

The close investigation of the homesickness syndrome has suggested that an appropriate conceptualisation is that of an hierarchical model of causal factors. Domination of cognition by home-related ruminations drives psychological distress, absent-mindedness and sub-optimum health. Although some attempt has been made to investigate the main theories of loss, interruption, role change or control loss, in terms of the particular symptoms of distress, the results cannot be conclusive. The rise in depression and obsessionality for *all* students might imply that the control hypothesis is supported. However, the interaction of anxiety with the transition for the homesick group might also imply that separation and loss, interruption and role models are also appropriate.

At this stage in the account of the causes of homesickness, it appears that we are moving towards a multi-causal approach in which both the pre- and post-transition environments have an important role to play in creating as well as maintaining the cognitive focus which in turn drives the symptoms. It would not be unreasonable to suppose that homesickness is a specific form of post-traumatic stress syndrome.

6

Circumstantial and Vulnerability Factors in Homesickness

The main difficulty with investigations of circumstantial and personal factors as influential variables, is that the decision as to which particular variables to include constrains the outcome. The technique of introducing a large range of variables and then identifying critical ones is not desirable (a) because this means lengthy questionnaires and subjects may be less likely to complete all of them adequately, and (b) because the technique capitalises on chance associations.

It was decided to take a theory-driven approach where possible, and to limit the number of variables included. In the first part of this chapter there is consideration of the role of personal factors such as involvement in the decision to go to school or university; satisfaction with the new environment; and desire for home visits. These factors may indicate the degree of personal control a person feels he or she has over the move. Personality factors such as self-esteem, depression and obsessionality, extraversion, and hysteria are also included in this section. In the second section, other circumstantial factors thought to be likely factors in the response to transition are described. These include geographical distance of the move, home background, and life history factors.

An interesting but unexpected finding is that when results of the university and boarding school studies were compared, some factors were influential in one context but not in the other. This might imply population-specific effects in that the minds of children are different in important respects from the minds of students. Or it might be a result of overall impact of life-style differences. These are the issues that are dealt with towards the end of this chapter. The issues serve to illustrate the importance of the context in which people live their lives and emphasise that stressful experiences occur in contexts which may help to shape the reaction of the individual.

PERSONAL FACTORS IN HOMESICKNESS REPORTING

Sex Differences

Few clear direct sex differences have been found in either the populations of school children, university students or student nurses. This is against informally held beliefs of laymen and professionals alike which indicate that females are more likely to feel homesick. Only in the context of the Australian boarding school in the Bush, studied by Fisher and Peacock, was there any indication that homesickness incidence was greater in females. The special conditions of the school with emphasis on hard physical exercise and general heavy work duties in maintaining school buildings and facilities might have had a greater adverse effect on girls and may account for this result.

In the context of the U.K. studies, the lack of sex differences in homesickness reporting becomes puzzling given the literature suggesting that females react with greater psychoneurotic symptoms (e.g. see Hood et al., 1987; Fisher & Hood, 1988). One possibility is that the distress in females is caused by factors other than the effects of separation from home. Perhaps the pressures to succeed in a new competitive academic environment provide sources of anxiety and distress, and the female students react by perseverance and struggle to succeed. This would fit with the finding from the Fisher & Hood studies showing that females also adapt better to university.

It was only possible to examine the age factor within the particular populations studied. In the school pupils this was 11–14 years; in the students it was 17–27 years. To combine groups in order to examine the age range would not be a valid process because, as will be shown later in the chapter, the school and university populations differed in many other respects.

Decisional Control Over the Move

Little information is available on how the decision to go to university is made. The decision to leave home for school is different in that for the schools studied, the pupil is enlisted early, sometimes even at birth and may have very little direct influence on his fate because of the authority of parents at this age. We found very few school pupils who felt that there was much personal control over the decision to go away to boarding school.

As indicated in earlier chapters, work on the perception of control as a moderating variable in stress (Fisher, 1984) suggests that having control over an event frequently lessens the threatening nature of that event. This is perhaps best illustrated by laboratory studies in animal and human populations where having control over unpleasant experiences such as shock, generally ameliorates the stressful effects. For animals this is manifest in terms of physical symptoms, whereas for human beings, tolerance is the most affected variable (see Fisher, 1986, Chapter 2).

The difficulties of defining control in a variety of different life situations makes extrapolation from laboratory to real life settings problematic; nevertheless it might be argued that a person would be less threatened by a move from home to attend an institution if there was control over the decision to go, if the university had been personally selected in the first place, or if there were positive reasons for wanting to go (as compared with being forced by family).

One reason would be that if there is high decisional involvement then there is self-selection in favour of those who want to go to university. If there is low decisional involvement then there may be willingness or unwillingness to make the transition. A second reason is that the act of taking the initiative may be a positive sign of willingness to become committed. There is of course the problem that the homesick might 'rewrite history' and perceive the decisions of the past differently when viewing them from the perspective of a distressed state. The possibility of such state-dependent distortions must be borne in mind.

Results from studies in which those reporting homesickness were asked to indicate on a category-rating scale the perceived level of responsibility for the decision to go to university, indicated that it was less for homesick as compared with non-homesick students (Fisher et al., 1985). However, there was no such effect for boarding school pupils. One interpretation is that school children generally do not expect to have much control over decisions affecting their lives because they are used to parental authority. Absence of decisional control might be more stressful at later stages in developmental history when the expectancy and need for operating control is greater.

Personal Satisfaction

Data from homesick university students (Fisher, 1985) showed that satisfaction with residence was lower for the homesick than for the non-homesick group. A similar effect has been reported by Kane (1987) in studies conducted in Manchester. The homesick group also were more pessimistic in their ratings of current friendships relative to previous friendships than non-homesick students, and indicated that they had expected better friendships. Overall, the data did not suggest dissatisfaction but rather a lack of the same level of satisfaction as indicated by the non-homesick.

Informally, one or two wardens of the university residences indicated that very often those who are homesick appear to have the less desirable rooms and more often than not are randomly allocated shared rooms. Perhaps some kind of cognitive evaluation of assets obtained and assets lost may create the preconditions for missing home. This is in line with the congruence model outlined in Chapter 2 and will be discussed further in later chapters. Perhaps what is needed is a computational model in which home and the new environment are weighed up in terms of the balance of comforts and challenges offered. University environments are more likely to be seen as challenging but low in comfort and security (made worse by small income grants); home offers less challenge and opportunity for expansion but more comfort and care-giving.

Personal Desire for Visits Home

Homesick students were found to indicate greater intensity of desire to make visits home than non-homesick students. There was also a positive correlation between the desire to go home and the frequency of homesickness reporting for those who reported homesickness ($r_s = 0.22; p < 0.05$). However, the reported desire in the homesickness group to go home more frequently was not actualised because the number of visits home in the first six weeks of term did not distinguish the homesick and non-homesick groups (data reported in Fisher, Murray, & Frazer, 1985). Perhaps the existence of the desire, but the lack of attempt to consummate it, represent important features of the homesick state. The homesick person may be locked into a conflict whereby he or she is forced to stay in the new environment because of the realisation that opportunities for the future are offered.

Personality Characteristics

Of those features examined, extraversion showed an association with homesickness reporting but this was a low correlation ($-0.19, p < 0.05$). Hysteria, on the Middlesex Hospital Questionnaire, also correlated negatively with homesickness reporting ($-0.31, p < 0.05$), and the non-homesick had consistently higher scores ($p < 0.03$). However hysteria has some special properties on the MHQ (see Crown & Crisp, 1966) and this makes interpretation difficult.

The hypothesis that low and high self-esteem do not distinguish reactions prior to a life event but do so after a life event, was examined in the context of a transition from home. No difference was found between self-esteem levels in homesick and non-homesick groups. However there was one interesting finding which may have confounded this effect; the Scottish students were found to have lower self-esteem than the students from England. We have no explanation as to why this should be the case. If anything, the English who come up to the Scottish universities often do so through the clearing house system because they have not qualified for their first choice; it might have been predicted that they would have had lower self-esteem. This issue clearly needs looking at again in greater detail and may be of interest to counsellors.

Trait factors cannot be distinguished from states of psychoneurotic symptoms which may be manifestations of current stress or vulnerability. Some evidence of personal vulnerability was found in the context of a longitudinal study by Fisher and Hood (1987). There were raised scores on the Middlesex Hospital Questionnaire and particularly on subscale scores depression and obsessionality prior to leaving home (see discussions in the last half of the previous chapter).

The Cognitive Failure Questionnaire also differentiated homesick and non-homesick students, indicating the former to be more absent-minded (Fisher et al., 1985). The degree to which cognitive failure is a trait with durable qualities (as proposed by Broadbent et al., 1982), or has state features is yet to be resolved (see Fisher & Hood, 1987; Reason, 1988). Cognitive failure level did not indicate vulnerability in that it did not predict the rise in psychoneurotic scores following the transition to university (Fisher & Hood, 1987).

The issue of the role of vulnerability factors in the response to life events is complex. Most studies of vulnerability focus on predisposing factors in early life history (e.g. see Brown, 1988). However there might also be precipitant-precipitant effects. Maybe an anxious year at school could predispose a person to react adversely to the transition to university. Thus, as envisaged in the original Holmes and Rahe (1965) research, life stresses may have additive properties which influence a common mechanism.

In the context of the above findings suggesting vulnerability to homesickness, the following explanations are possible: (1) the person later to be homesick, anticipates the threat of the impending move and is already reacting with depression; (2) the person later to be homesick, is vulnerable to the effects of the transition because of the effects of the demands of the last year at school; (3) the person later to be homesick has trait depression characteristics and is likely to react adversely both to leaving home and to the idea of commitment to the new environment.

With regard to (3) above, there is an interesting issue concerning depression and commitment. Depression is generally associated with loss of volition and apathy. This would lead to the prediction that becoming committed to any person or place would be difficult. However, Kuhl and Kazen-Saad (1988) have argued that the problem for the depressed might be the de-activation of intention when a goal proves non-attainable. This would suggest that the depressed do not lack the ability to become commited but they lack the ability to disengage from a previous commitment. Thus in the context of the discussions on vulnerability to homesickness, it may be the case that the potentially homesick may be unable to release commitments to established home routines. This should be a non-adaptive position with regard to transitions; the depressed should be poor movers and should be slow to adapt to change.

SITUATIONAL CONTEXTS AND HOMESICKNESS REPORTING

Geographical Distance

A situational factor of importance is geographical distance. There are two reasons for predicting that it might be influential. First, the greater the distance incurred the greater the liklihood of change in culture—hence the greater the liklihood of culture shock. Secondly, the greater the distance incurred the greater the possibility that the individual will feel cut off from home and unable to visit it. The financial cost of long distance telephone calls or journeys home could prove daunting for a student on a low financial budget. There is also cost in terms of time for long journeys, especially if this is to be done on a limited financial budget and involves, for example, hitch-hiking.

Fisher et al., 1985 reported the results of a study in which the frequency of homesickness was indicated on a category-rating scale from 'never' through to 'extremely frequent'. The scale therefore afforded a measure of incidence 'never' as compared with the other frequency categories, and also afforded a measure of level of frequency. The results for incidence showed that for university students, distance from home distinguished homesick and non-homesick groups. The average distance from home for the homesick group was 364 miles, whereas the average distance for the non-homesick group was 203 miles. This was significantly different ($p < 0.05$); although the distance was not large it is large within the U.K. context.

The frequency measure of homesickness reporting in the homesick groups was not distinguished by geographical distance. This suggested that geographical distance could be assumed to operate as an initiating rather than an augmenting factor.

No particular home locations were identified for homesick students. There was no evidence to suggest that they were from rural or urban locations. There was no indication to suggest that they were English rather than Scottish students (defined by current home location). The 'culture shock' explanation assumes the effect to be due to the difference in local custom, habits, language, and so on. Dundee is a working-class town and although in a scenic setting on the estuary of the River Tay, it would present a student from the south of England with a different cultural experience. Speech characteristics are different and for the English student local dialects may be sometimes difficult to follow. Public houses are more austere. There is Sunday opening of shops and Scotland has a different religious background (Presbyterian). However since there was no evidence for preponderance of English (relative to percentage intake of English to the University) in the homesick group, the culture shock hypothesis was not supported.

The alternative explanation is that geographical distance affects the probability of home visits because of financial costs (important to a limited-income student) and because of the time involved. One result of importance is that homesick and non-homesick students did not differ in the number of visits home; therefore any effect of distance must be due to perceived isolation rather than the amelioration produced by actual home visits by the non-homesick.

An unexpected result was that there is no effect of geographical distance on the homesickness reporting of boarding school children, although the range of distance involved was comparable with that of the students (Fisher et al., 1986). This intriguing result provides a further hint that factors which are operative for one population are not necessarily operative for another. In the case of boarding school children, visits home tend to be limited and organised; therefore geographical distance cannot affect the probability of a home visit. Moreover, the public schools draw from a wealthy socioeconomic catchment and therefore financial costs are less likely to be influential. These considerations indicate the importance of general life contexts as determinants of the influence of specific situational variables.

Taken collectively, the results indicate that it is the feeling of being distanced and removed from home that is influential but only when home-visiting remains a possibility. Thus the student could go home and may witness his colleagues who live near to home doing so; the school pupil is rarely faced with the dilemma because visits home are not under personal discretion. Perhaps for the student at university, having the potential for visits home but with great cost penalties for long distance visits creates a state of conflict. By contrast the school pupil has been used to parental authority and is protected from experiencing too much control over important decisions too early. Absence of the possibility of visits home prevents decisional conflict.

These issues need further exploration because of the practical import-ance for those dealing with the homesick. An obvious question is whether home visits should be encouraged initially or whether it is better to force the student to become adapted to the new life by discouraging contact with home. It could be argued that visits home would be highly disruptive and would merely rekindle any unhappiness on return to the new environment. By analogy with the bereaved were it possible to allow them to visit the deceased occasionally it could be expected that the experience of grief would recur after each visit.

Home Background and Life History

No evidence has been found to suggest that birth order, number of siblings, parental harmony, or parental loss (by death or divorce) are factors in homesickness in either school or student populations. Unexpectedly, a study of school pupils showed that having a sibling already established at the school did not influence homesickness reporting but tended to act as a stress factor; pupils reported feelings of being under scrutiny, being more subject to teasing, and having to live up to expectations and standards set by the already established sibling (Fisher et al., 1984; 1986).

The main methodological problem in examining the life history of the homesick is that there was found to be a reporting bias towards reporting positive aspects of previous life history. This is logically consistent with missing and grieving for home but creates difficulties for the collection of data about life history from retrospective report.

In the diaries presented to boarding school pupils, a page was devoted to collecting life history data. A single line marked off in age units was presented and respondents indicated by arrows, happy/positive events on the left and unhappy/negative events on the right. The order of completing the entries was indicated by numbers—'1' against the first event; '2' against the second event etc. It was found that homesick subjects reported more positive events first, suggesting that there may be a valence factor in cognition concerning representation of 'home' and previous life history events.

The finding that recall of life events reflects properties of current state is well established in the research literature on life events and illness. In the research literature on, for example, life events and coronary heart disease, the phrase 'effort after meaning' is sometimes used to describe the tend-ency of cardiac patients to make sense of a disorder frequently associated with stress and thus to over-report stressful events in immediate life history (see Boman, 1988). There is also experimental evidence to suggest that mood states influence recall properties. The depressed are more likely to recall unpleasant life events and may be faster to recall them (see Lloyd &

Lishman, 1975; Rapaport, 1961). Therefore the finding of no association of homesickness with negative life events in history has to be considered with some caution. Any effect may be swamped by a reporting bias in favour of home.

SITUATIONAL FACTORS AND THE COMPETING DEMANDS MODEL

Population-specific Effects

As described above, where it has proved possible to obtain comparable measures of variables in both school and university populations, there is some evidence to suggest that there are effects which are population-specific. For example, geographical distance is a factor in homesickness for university students whereas it is not influential in school populations. The same is true for decisional control over the transition; it differentiates the homesick and non-homesick populations at university but not at boarding school.

The generality of this finding could not be checked on all measures of distress (especially those of mental health and psychoneuroticism), because of the constraints imposed by the schools on what could be assessed. However, there is a hint that *different total life contexts* themselves influence which variables differentiate the homesick and non-homesick groups.

The Competing Demands Model and Homesickness

The competing demands model, as developed in Chapter 4, provides a conceptual framework for understanding how and why thoughts of home dominate thinking and are associated with distress. The model could be described in hydraulic terms because the important feature is that home thoughts compete to dominate the attention mechanism but may be attenuated when the person becomes committed to the new environment because other sources of information become dominant. Thus, the person who 'engages' the environment and becomes active may perhaps inadvertently control his or her tendency to be homesick.

Homesickness could thus be sustained as much by a failure to become committed as by a chronic threat caused by loss of immediate contact with home. The difference between episodic reporters and non-episodic reporters may be in terms of the ability to allow the new environment to provide effective competition with homesick thoughts rather than with the intensity of the effects of separation from home.

From the results described in this chapter it appears that there are both personal and situational factors which operate to influence homesickness reporting and that *different total life style and contexts* might decide which are likely to be operative. Thus decisional control is only influential for students because by that age, responsibility is expected and therefore not to have control is threatening (or that self-selection did not occur). It is not influential for boarding school children because parental authority dominates and control is not expected. Equally, increased geographical distance creates a feeling of being isolated for those students who retain the option to visit home but find it costly to do so, but does not operate for school children who are restricted to the school environment by the rules imposed.

How do we integrate such results with the competing demands model? There are three possibilities. The first is that these population-specific factors act directly to influence the degree of distress experienced on leaving home. This seems unlikely because there is no evidence that the low control life-style of the children at school increases homesickness incidence, frequency, or duration as compared with the high control student groups. A second possibility is that these factors are influential in both populations but that circumstantial factors can attenuate their influence. This is in fact what is represented in Fig. 6.1. Thirdly, we may be dealing with some complex self-selection differences; students with more responsibility for the decisions may be more able to self-select than the school children. On the assumption that self-selection means that those who are less likely to be distressed make the transition, this might also imply less homesickness reporting in the student group, and this is found not to be the case.

Figure 6.1 illustrates the most plausible possibility, namely that the impact of separation and loss may be influenced by situational factors, especially those which concern being able to reverse the situation (control) or being able to remain in close contact with home (visits and so on). However, specific life-style contexts in the new environment determine whether these factors can operate to influence distress. The difference in school and university populations means that these factors are neither necessary nor sufficient conditions, but act as moderators.

Perhaps the most likely explanation is that an hierarchical model of influence is required. As illustrated in Fig. 6.1, total life context can act as a 'gate device' overruling the effect of a number of moderator variables thus creating population-specific effects. The figure also illustrates the possibility that variables may act at different stages of the homesick-induction process. Separation and loss and interruption are activated by the transition from home and the impact may be made more threatening by low ability to reverse the situation or by high cost of trying to maintain direct home contacts. By contrast, personal vulnerability may act later in the process to influence the ability of a person to create competing thoughts through environmental commitment.

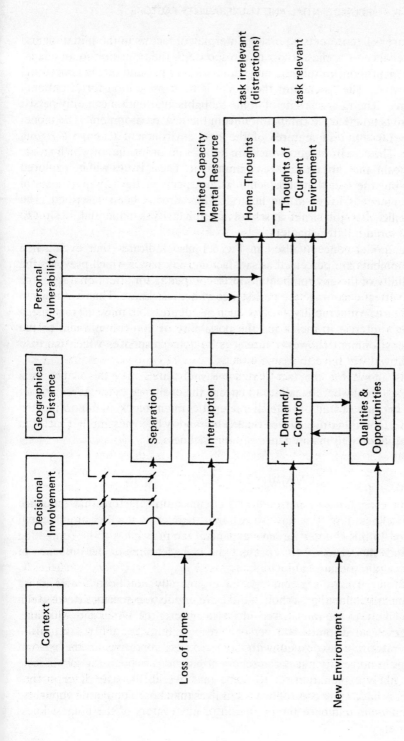

FIG. 6.1. Competing demands model: Homesickness imagery competes with environmental demands for mental resource.

77

Figure 6.1 represents a possible interplay of factors in the initiation and maintenance of homesickness as a response to the transition to an educational institution. In subsequent chapters we try to build on the conceptual framework. The essence of the model is the competition for attentional resource. The raised profile of home thoughts in attention can only persist if there is no effective competition from the new environment. The model allows for different features of the new environment to have a strong effect. Thus environments which are unpleasant or hostile, or which create 'job strain' may not encourage commitment. These issues will be explored later, but the fact that satisfaction with aspects of the new psychosocial environment is lower in the homesick has already been described. The possibility that 'job strain' at school and university is influential, has yet to be explored in later chapters.

The model conceptualised in Fig. 6.1 also indicates that even when environments are perceived as satisfactory, any factor which prevents the possibility of the environmental source competing for attentional resource will in effect encourage the persistence of homesickness. Thus as shown in the figure, vulnerability factors such as depression may act against a person's interest in increasing the possibility of non-commitment to the new environment (however nice it is). Phobic responses which increase withdrawal will have the same effect.

This allows for the fact that some individuals may be caught in a feedback loop whereby failure to engage the challenge of the new environment because of trait or state characteristics might block an important step in the adaptation process. Personal vulnerability becomes another factor in the initiation and maintenance of homesickness.

SUMMARY AND CONCLUSIONS

The investigations of personal and circumstantial factors that influence homesickness reporting have shown that there are a number of influential factors. In this chapter we have expanded the principles of the competing demands model to try to represent the main features of the influence of personal and situational factors.

Factors such as sex and age have generally not been found to be particularly influential, although there are population-specific effects which seem likely to be due to the life-style differences associated with age. Geographical distance and personal responsibility for the transition are each positively associated with homesickness reporting in the student groups at university but not in school populations in boarding school. The most likely explanation seems to be that overall life-style is important; students have more control over their lives than boarding school pupils and these factors influence the operation of moderators of the homesickness experience.

The new environment may play an important role, in that commitment can be encouraged if it is seen to be desirable and enjoyable. Conversely, hostile or unpleasant environments are likely to have the reverse effect. We would predict that leaving home to take a much longed for holiday in a pleasant environment is less likely to create homesickness than leaving home to begin work in an educational institution.

However, even if the environment is pleasant and offers what is desired, those who are prone to depression or phobic reactions may for a number of reasons fail to become committed and therefore fail to generate the competing information which will help to attentuate homesick thoughts. Thus personal vulnerability factors may operate to determine whether or not homesickness continues or is attentuated.

The model presented in this chapter is partly a descriptive formulation portraying what we believe to be the interplay of a number of complex circumstantial and personal factors in the experience of homesickness. At the heart of the formulation is the notion of competition for attentional resource. The break with home provides one source which competes for attention; the new environment provides challenge and new sources of information which can compete effectively. It is the progress and resolution of conflict that is assumed to be influential in determining the process of adaptation and the reduction of distress.

7 Thinking Homesick: The Implications of Differences in Cognitive Organisation and Memory

In the previous chapters, the origins of homesick thoughts have been hypothesised to be associated with the effects of loss, separation, interruption, or role change. In each case, the issue of whether the psychological state of the homesick is quantitatively or qualitatively different from that of the non-homesick is a relevant issue. If the homesick are assumed to be quantitatively different from the non-homesick this might be because the impact of loss, interruption, or role change, is greater, producing a more profound effect. Alternatively the homesick might be qualitatively different because of the organisation of cognitive structures. Perhaps, for example, a nervous system structured to focus on the past (nostalgic) is associated with different impact when loss or interruption occurs.

This chapter is concerned with considering the cognitive state of the homesick. Issues of theoretical interest concern the dominance of home-orientated thoughts and whether the homesick differ quantitatively or qualitatively in terms of cognitive factors.

On first consideration, an efficient planning system should be organised in such a way as to ensure that plans which are dominant in the nervous system are those which are appropriate to the occasion. In other words, there should be control over which plans are in focus. The person who drives his car whilst his attention is dominated by a plan directing action sequences for shopping in a supermarket would be at risk for accidents. Domination of the planning system by inappropriate plans of the past could effectively reduce control of planned activity.

It appears that the bereaved and the homesick as well as those distressed by a life experience are dominated by intrusive information from the past.

A planning system which allows this to happen could be argued to be ineffective and does not favour change. On the other hand, perhaps as argued by Fisher (1984), reflective 'regurgitation' of the past may provide the means whereby the routines of the past can be incorporated into new plans. During the 'integration' period, the domination of thoughts from the past may be a side-effect or epiphenomenon. Perhaps those people who are nostalgic are those who have a more efficient planning mechanism and are more adaptive in the long term.

BACKGROUND ISSUES IN PLANNED ACTIVITY

A fundamental change in the way human behaviour was considered to be organised was provided by Miller, Galanter, and Pribram (1960). They proposed that behaviour is organised with consequence in mind, is hierarchically structured in the form of a plan or blueprint in the nervous system, and involves a sequential series of decisions. Miller et al. provided a conceptualisation of the blueprint for behaviour in terms of the TOTE unit, which represents four elements of decision making: (1) 'Test' whereby reality is contrasted with what is desired; (2) 'Operate' whereby action to resolve any discrepancy evident at the test phase is selected; (3) 'Test' whereby the initial test element is repeated; and (4) 'Exist' whereby if the discrepancy no longer exists behaviour is stable.

Figure 7.1 illustrates the essential nature of the TOTE unit. The example provided by Miller is that of hitting a nail into a piece of wood. Each 'test' phase which results in a discrepancy between reality (nail not flush with the wood) and desire (make nail flush with wood) results in an operation (striking nail with hammer) until the nail is finally flush with the wood. In turn, the operating phase (striking the nail with the hammer) itself involves a TOTE unit. Thus blueprints become selected by the operating phase of larger blueprints and TOTE units are organised in an embedded way.

Contained in this analysis are two essential ingredients for purposeful behaviour. The first is the 'state of the world' or reality; the second is the intention which is assumed to relate to overall ambition. Thus a person perceives the state of a particular world, conceives of how he or she would like the world to be, and selects a set of actions for reducing the discrepancy. Fisher (1984) proposed this process of discrepancy reduction as the basis of cognitive representation of control. A memory representation which provided evidence of successive discrepancy reduction would indicate that control was not possible.

If it is envisaged that the blueprints for a variety of skills and behaviours are available in memory such that they can be called up when needed, the

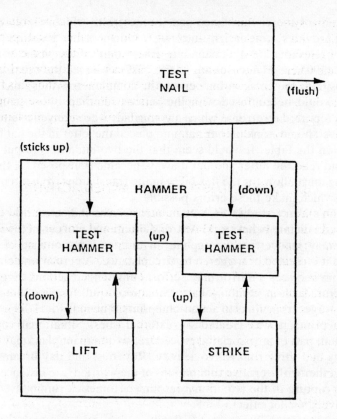

FIG. 7.1.   The hierarchical plan for hammering nails. Redrawn from Miller, Galanter, and Pribram (1960), with the permission of the authors and Holt, Rinehart and Winston.

implication is that they must be stored in an organised way, with locations in memory which can be addressed by the two ingredients: intention and reality. Storage should facilitate ready access to appropriate plans; the organism which can retrieve an appropriate blueprint for prevailing circumstance is best equipped for survival.

A contribution to understanding planning has been made by researchers concerned with features of human error. Errors might be conceived of as faults in the planning process resulting in actions not as intended (see Reason, 1988). They will almost certainly create conditions of transient loss of control; the man who attempts to deal with an immediate threat by faulty action can become caught in a feedback loop whereby outcome is increasingly decided by external factors (see Fisher, 1984, Chapter 7).

Analysis of the circumstance and the descriptive features of cognitive failures provides some insight into the workings of the planning process, and is of relevance for understanding absent-mindedness in the homesick. Jastrow (1905) and later Reason (1976, 1977) observed the occurrences of transposition or 'cross-wiring' errors in complex activities; one set of actions would be confused with the actions required by a second task. Jastrow reported an error in which a young lady who received a letter when she arrived home, took off her hat, and placed the letter in the hat box and the hat on the table. It would seem that the two intentions to put the hat away and read the letter and put it away, became transposed. A theory of planning must allow for the flexibility in the translations from intentions to actions which make these errors possible.

Reason's diary studies of human errors have indicated how circumstances can dictate behaviours. A strong situational pull can occur so that a person may inadvertently complete an unintended sequence of actions because it is created or triggered by circumstance. A person who enters the bathroom and sees a mirror may perform unintended actions triggered by the mirror, such as combing hair. 'Situational pull' implies that circumstances forge strong links to action-blueprints. The individual did not select the blueprint; it was created by external cues. Situational cues may implement part of an associated procedure, so dominant plans may capture thoughts and drive ruminative activity. Reveries, and day dreams of the old, together with negative ruminations of the worried, are instances where there is capture of the attentional resource. Homesick ruminative activity may have a similar effect.

LOSS, TRANSITION, AND PLAN RUNNING

Faults in Plan Running

If the response to loss and separation creates a mental state dominated by ruminations with content from the pre-loss or pre-transition environment, this raises factors of interest for a theory of the planning of human behaviour. It could be argued that this is not an obvious organisational aspect of daily planned behaviour; a person does not normally become dominated by recent events. If he completes the process of cooking a meal he does not sit eating the meal, mentally dominated by the plans involved in preparing it. The planning process needs to be organised in such a way that plans are switched in and out of focus and in accordance with requirements.

There are two conditions, however, in which the transference of plans might become altered: the first is if the task is interrupted. The interruption model as proposed by Mandler and colleagues (Mandler, 1975) allows for the dominance in cognition of thwarted or interrupted plans. The second condition which might have similar consequences is the occurrence of an error, particularly one which results in an accident. Claparede's law of awareness (Claparede, 1934) was originally formulated to describe the effect of an accident on an actor during the performance of a play; the actor would become distracted by the event and aware of reality rather than the acting role.

One possibility is that planning structure allows for the switching in of cognitive material which is of a highly pertinent or emotional nature. An alternative, first considered by Fisher (1984) is that the planning system is organised in such a way that 'regurgitation' of plans following a specified event is made possible in order that new conceptual frameworks and new plans can be formulated and refined.

The Domination of Home Thoughts

Many subjects in the studies, reported informally that a routine activity such as taking a bath or going to a well-known chain store would trigger thoughts of home, but in addition could evoke images of inappropriate plans. A person taking a bath in a new residence might reach out for a towel using directives associated with the location of a bath towel at home. The act of waking up in the morning would sometimes create moments of confusion because the sleeper would think he or she was in bed at home. One suggestion is that home-related activity is dominant in memory and is therefore easily triggered by circumstance.

The dominance of home thoughts in the minds of those who recently moved, was indicated by a study (reported in Chapter 5) in which self-reported 'home' and 'school' problems and associated periods of worry and preoccupation were examined using a diary style presentation, in boarding school children (Fisher et al., 1984). Analysis of percentage reports of different categories of problems as classified by the investigators, showed that although more school problems were reported as compared with home-orientated problems, the latter were found to be associated with greater periods of worrying. Thus the problem/worry ratios effectively distinguished school and home orientated problem classes, illustrating the mind-grabbing superiority of home affairs.

There could be a number of reasons for this. First, it might be the case that leaving home creates new problems (e.g. concern about leaving parents, pets and so on). Secondly, it might be the case that ongoing home problems persist and are less controllable because of the increased distance. Some recent studies in other occupational settings have indicated that worrying is more likely for occupational problems which have low control (see Fisher, 1987). Finally, it is possible that a move creates compulsive ruminative activity and routine plans dominate cognition.

An issue of importance is whether the same thought content prevails for homesick and non-homesick subjects. This addresses the idea of whether homesickness is qualitatively or quantitatively different from non-homesickness in terms of the content of home-related cognitive activity. Discussions in previous chapters have assumed that the difference is quantitative rather than qualitative.

Plan Running in the Homesick

An issue of interest therefore concerns the nature of home-related thoughts in the homesick as compared with the non-homesick. Could it be the case that those who are homesick have more problems to contend with (either ongoing problems, such as health of parents, or newly created problems due to leaving home, such as care of a pet), and that homesickness really only represents the need to go home and cope with existing problems? If this is the case then what we are really indicating is that non-homesick and homesick subjects differ qualitatively in the content of their home-related thinking because the homesick have more pertinent and demanding home-related problems to contend with.

This section is prefaced by the point that since investigation of thought content of individuals depends on self-report, it is by definition highly subjective and many of the normally accepted checks are not possible. It may even be the case that the homesick justify their mental state of distress by the kind of data they report. In spite of these difficulties, it was thought useful to try to gain some impression of the likely content of home thoughts in the homesick and the non-homesick.

The study involved 47 subjects who provided definitions of homesickness (as described in previous chapters) and were found not to be differentiated by the definitions of homesickness which they provided. Subjects were first-year university students tested in the sixth week of the first term, and indicated their levels of homesickness on a five-category frequency scale from 'not homesick' through to 'extremely homesick'. They were then divided into homesick and non-homesick groups by partitioning scores on the scale into the zero category compared with categories 1–4. This dichotomy resulted in incidence of 63% homesickness reports.

Subjects were then asked to indicate on a pre-prepared set of scales, the proportion of time in which home-orientated thoughts were concerned with: (1) problems specifically created by leaving home; (2) ongoing problems (defined as problems already in existence prior to leaving home); and (3) uncontrollable home imagery (defined as intrusive thoughts about home routine and locations).

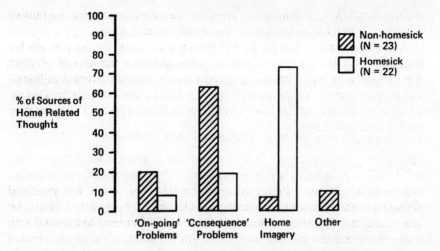

FIG. 7.2.   Self-reported classes of home ruminations in students.

As illustrated by Fig. 7.2, it was found that uncontrollable imagery predominated for the homesick (73%), whereas problems created by leaving home predominated for the non-homesick (63%). The difference in the proportions of thought-types reported for each of the two groups was significant on a Friedman Two-Way Analysis of Variance ($0.05 > p < 0.01$) for each group. Specific comparisons confirmed the between-group differences in the proportion of home-problems, consequence-problems and intrusive imagery in that the homesick reported significantly more home imagery and significantly less of either type of home problems.

This finding was further investigated with a set of 39 students, 25 of whom reported homesickness. The students were asked to write down examples of the sort of home-orientated thoughts they had. The written statements were also classified by each student in terms of the following labels: 'uncontrolled imagery'; problems ongoing at the time of leaving home; and problems created by leaving home.

The results showed that the homesick reported more imagery of home and family: 'I imagine myself going up to my room'; 'I think of myself sitting watching television with Mum and Dad'; 'Seems funny but I spend a lot of my time there—at home—in my head'; 'I walk about there, take the dog out, clean the car, take a bath; I do it during lectures and make myself upset'.

Statements containing one or more statement of imagery (as defined above) were produced by 85% of homesick students but only 12% of non-homesick students. Conversely, the non-homesick students were more concerned with problems at home: 'I hope my mother's leg is healing and that she is managing without me' (ongoing problem); 'Whether the dog is taken out. I hope he doesn't fret. I miss the cuddles' (problem created by leaving home). These accounted for 71% of the reported thoughts of non-homesick students but 15% for homesick students. (The percentages do not add up to 100 because they are based on scores in each of the available categories.)

The Regurgitation Model of Planning in the Homesick

The above accounts, although highly subjective, provide some hints about the nature of plan running processes. Fisher (1984) argued that domination of attention by plans of the past represents a rather inefficient planning process because resources would be swamped by inappropriate plans for action and the organism should have low survival value. In evolutionary terms, focus on the present and future should be more beneficial. However, it was counter-argued that there might be certain benefits to reflective activity involving old plans. The main benefit would be that it provides a means of consolidating past information and thus benefiting from experiences. An organism which is able to benefit from past experience should be at an evolutionary advantage. 'Regurgitation' sessions would permit full records of moves and countermoves, or even bad moves, and consequences to be established in cognition. Networks which represent possible and actual levels of controllability established during various stages of life experience could be consolidated.

Seen in this light, homesickness would be an adaptive state of reflection and regurgitation; the homesick should eventually adapt better to a new environment following transition. Unfortunately, we have no evidence to support this. If anything, the reverse appears to be supported by the data; the homesick show poorer scores on Crombag's College Adaptation Questionnaire (Crombag 1968; Fisher & Hood 1987).

However, university and school environments may be rather artificial environments because so much is demanded of a new pupil or student within the early weeks of arrival. The pupil or student needs to be alert, active and information seeking. Regurgitation of the past could interfere with the demands of coping with the new environment because of overload of the resource. Even if reflective preoccupation with the past eventually benefits adaptation, it will be disadvantageous in the early stages in that it could overload resources and create withdrawal. Thus, commitment to the new environment could be impaired. Structured cognitive activity in which regurgitation of the past is controlled would seem to combine the benefits of allowing the past to continue to influence the future and at the same time, not allowing it to attenuate commitment.

One hypothesis is that the homesick are operating a highly adaptive mechanism but that in the particular context of being simultaneously exposed to a new, highly demanding environment, it does not pay off and in fact produces secondary problems. Perhaps in evolutionary perspective, the nervous system was structured for accomplishing transitions to new environments with similar characteristics to the previous environments and where sudden step-function change in demand was not apparent.

MEMORY CHARACTERISTICS OF THE HOMESICK

Psychological State and Memory

There is a growing research literature which suggests that psychological state influences the organisation and retrieval of information. It would not be possible within the confines of this book to attempt a detailed review of state-dependent learning effects. The main issue of interest is whether the homesick differ from the non-homesick in the recall of current and pre-transition experiences.

Of particular interest is whether there is evidence of an 'hedonic set' determining the way the homesick view the past as compared with the current environment. It would seem that the very nature of homesickness assumes that home is desired and seen in positive terms. On the other hand, the existence of increased depressed symptoms in the homesick might suggest that recall even of aspects of home should be negative. If the latter alternative is true it would then seem strange that the homesick are obsessed with a past that they perceive in negative terms.

Studies which are laboratory-based have looked at the content and speed of recall of pleasant and unpleasant information (see Rapaport, 1961). Clinical studies of depressed and anxious patients have indicated that the depressed provide negative content to ideations and dreams, whereas the anxious provide threat-relevant content (Beck, 1967; 1970). The depressed, for example, seem relatively fast to produce negative thoughts and slow to produce positive thoughts relative to their non-depressed counterparts. Although laboratory studies often involve effects of marginal significance there is some support for this hypothesis (e.g. see Lloyd & Lishman, 1975). The existence of pessimistic bias in the depressed is of importance because of negative influence on recall of life events.

Dominant Features of Memory in the Homesick

A possible explanation of the apparent dominance of the cognition of the homesick by intrusive ideations of home, is that home thoughts occupy dominant positions in memory and are accessed first at times of distress.

A pilot study involving 35 first year students, 20 of whom were homesick and 15 of whom were not (from scores on a five-category rating scale), showed that when asked for a positive experience of home or university, the homesick were faster than the non-homesick to produce a verbal utterance of either a home thought or a university thought. However, content analysis of the thoughts produced suggested that the homesick were recalling essentially positive thoughts of home whereas the non-homesick reported a higher level of negative thoughts. There were more items with negative content produced by the homesick concerning university. This suggested that valence of recall differentiates the memory of homesick and non-homesick students.

Figure 7.3 shows the result of a study in which 30 non-homesick subjects who were in their third and fourth years at university and who scored greater than 9 on the Beck Depression Inventory (see Beck, 1967; 1970), were compared with a group of 36 first-year subjects who reported home-sickness (on a five-category rating scale) but scored less than 9 on the Beck Depression Inventory. Both groups were compared with a group of 21 control first-year subjects scoring less than 9 on the Beck Depression Inventory and zero homesickness incidence on the rating scale.

A between-group design was used to prevent difficulties associated with transfer or range effects. Each of the three groups was further sub-divided so that one sub-group of each was asked to produce either a negative or a positive thought of home. A second sub-group was asked to produce a negative or a positive thought concerning university. In effect this meant that there were 12 sub-groups and each subject only produced one re-sponse (or thought).

The method of recording elapsed time involved use of a voice key so that time from a signal to the subject's first utterance could be recorded. Examples of positive thoughts of university included: 'joining a sailing club'; 'my first lecture'; 'buying a university scarf'; 'having coffee with a group after a tutorial'; 'hill walking on Saturday'. Typical negative thoughts were: 'confusion in lecture'; 'hall food'; 'not having enough money'; 'having a great load of work in the first week'; 'no privacy in my room'. Non-parametric analysis of speed of recall of negative or positive thoughts of university showed that the depressed and homesick were not distinguished from each other: both groups differed from the control group.

Therefore, as shown in the figure, the results indicated that when generating thoughts of university, the homesick behaved very like the depressed in that they were slow to produce a positive example and fast to produce a negative example.

However, the homesick behaved differently from the depressed when asked to generate thoughts of home: The homesick were faster to have

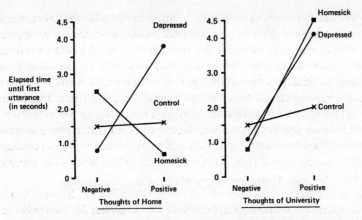

FIG. 7.3.   'Hedonic set' in the memory characteristics of homesick students.

positive thoughts but slower to have negative thoughts as compared with either the depressed or control groups. Examples of positive thoughts of home included: 'having breakfast with Mum and Dad'; 'going to my bedroom'; 'playing my records'; 'going out with the dog'; 'food'; 'hot drinks at night'; 'friends next door'. Examples of negative thoughts included: 'Mother nagging'; 'having to conform to set hours'; 'tidying room'; 'not allowed to play records loudly'; 'Father is out of work again'.

Thus the picture which emerges is that whereas the depressed appear to have a memory structure which facilitates unpleasant thoughts and memories *irrespective of environment*, for the homesick the facility is contingent on the focus of recall. Valence appears for the homesick to be structured with respect to environmental contingencies. There are important implications for understanding the organisation of memory for life experiences. However, it is impossible to know from these data whether the homesick have had a better time whilst growing up at home or whether the impact of university drives them to perceive home positively.

The finding of a differential valence in the memory of the homesick could give some support to the idea that the homesick have reveries of home because of their perceived pleasantness or in order to escape from reality. Perhaps there is addiction to the comforts and security of home: to give it up is to create unhappiness; to restore the experience by reverie offers some comfort even if there is the later penalty of distress.

The analogy with addiction is best illustrated in terms of the heroin addict who changes to methodone but then finds methodone less satisfactory in a number of ways; heroin therefore remains more attractive and the need for it dominates thinking. Perhaps the 'home-addict' is weaned off home and onto the new university environment but finds the new experience less acceptable. Thoughts of home (preferred), therefore begin to dominate thoughts. The latter argument would assume that some sort of value-weighting takes place as the individual assesses the benefits of the new environment against those of home. Universities and schools make considerable demands on students and it may be that it is the assessment of the 'home' as compared with the 'university' (or school) milieu that makes the basis of the discomfort and distress. Thus, leaving home for a much desired holiday might be totally different from leaving home to attend an institution for educational or vocational reasons.

HOMESICK THOUGHTS: A REAPPRAISAL

This chapter has been concerned with the features of the thinking and memory characteristics of the homesick. There are two issues of import- ance in that they provide further clues concerning the nature of the homesick response. First, as indicated initially, the thoughts of the home- sick, although centred on home, do not appear to be driven by problems which are ongoing or which are created by leaving home. This contrasts with non-homesick subjects who appear to direct more of their home- related thoughts to problems pre-existing or arising from the transition. There is thus a qualitative difference in the nature of cognitive activity in homesick and non-homesick subjects.

One possibility is that the dominance of intrusive home thoughts is purely mechanical. In other words, plans are so organised in the homesick that thoughts of the past are dominant. Running these plans may be distressing and their dominance creates the nostalgic thinker.

However, there is also the finding that there is positive valence attached to the organisation of home thoughts in the memory of the homesick. An explanation that takes account of this is that the apparent dominance of home thoughts is not mechanical but is strategic. Individuals seek home thoughts because home is such a desirable place and provides escape from reality. If the strategic explanation is valid, this suggests that the homesick are behaving as 'hedonists' retaining a mental commitment to home because it is infinitely preferable to developing commitments in the new environment. This may imply that some cognitive evaluation takes place within the first few weeks of the new term and that increasingly during this period of the evaluation, a negative result accrues—home is seen as more desirable because of security, comforts offered, or because of the support- ing and loving relationships with family and friends. An active hedonistic strategy of 'mental visits' to home produces benefits for the individual but of course creates the cost of recreating and maintaining the pain of separation. The penalty of nostalgia may be increased risk of distressing emotions and failure to adapt to university.

Finally, it might be that the intention to give up and return home triggers constant preoccupation with thoughts of home. The imagery would be positive and would reflect the state of decision making concerning action. The positive valence attached to home thoughts would be expected in circumstances where a person was actively selecting to return home as an option. The decision to go or stay might be the outcome of conflict involving protracted decision making in which the benefits and discomforts of staying are weighed against the benefits and cost's of leaving. During this time, dominance of home thoughts would be expected to determine cognition and to drive feelings of distress.

SUMMARY AND CONCLUSIONS

Examination of aspects of the structure of cognitive activity in the home-sick has differentiated them from non-homesick individuals in two essential respects. First, the evidence suggests that there is domination by intrusive home imagery in the homesick, whereas in the non-homesick, home directed thoughts are more directly concerned with problems. This indicates that there is a qualitatively different aspect of the content of cognitive activity in the homesick.

The second respect in which the homesick and non-homesick differ is in terms of the valence of home and university thoughts in cognition. It appears that the homesick function much like the depressed when providing instances of pleasant or unpleasant aspects of university life, in that they are fast to have unpleasant thoughts and slow to have pleasant thoughts.

However, when it comes to thinking of instances from the pre-transition or home environment, the homesick are fast to produce pleasant memories and slow to produce unpleasant memories. This again suggests that a qualitatively different aspect of cognitive organisation in the homesick is involved.

There are four possible explanations of these findings. The first is the structural explanation and implies that the homesick have cognitive structures which favour domination of the immediate past. They are nostalgic thinkers and are less likely to become enthusiastic and committed in new environments because they remain committed to the previous environments. They are thus likely to be poorly adapted to moves. The second explanation is that the homesick are like drug addicts deprived of a drug and constantly preoccupied with it during the early stage of what could be termed 'home-withdrawal'. Thirdly, the domination by thoughts of home might be a form of escapism. Reveries into the pleasantries of the past may be a way of avoiding current unhappiness. On this view, homesick ruminations arise strategically rather than mechanically.

Finally, it might be the case that concentration on thoughts of home is an epiphenomenon associated with the decision making which reviews the intention to leave and go home. The individual is lost in reveries concerned with home as the conflict takes place about the costs and benefits of going home as compared with staying.

8 Homesickness, Commitment, and the Job Strain Model

In all previous analyses, the role of the new environment in influencing homesickness has been envisaged in terms of the provision of competing information which attenuates homesick ruminations. The implication is that the new environment provides information sources which create effective competition for attentional resources. This analysis means that the new environment plays a moderating role in homesickness experience. It implies that environments which provide either conditions of challenge, or involve desirable features (as might be the case for holiday environments) are good attenuators of homesickness experience.

However more detailed consideration suggests that the important factor is commitment. Environmental properties can encourage but not determine commitment. In this chapter an interactional model is developed in which the nature of the individual and the nature of the new environment jointly determine commitment and thus jointly determine the level of moderation of homesickness experience.

Little is known about the process of commitment although its links with mental health have been explored. Klinger (1975) denotes 'current concern' as a state of sensitivity to a problem that has an onset (commitment) and an off-set (consummation or disengagement). A progression of initial commitment leading eventually to disengagement is assumed to be accompanied by mood changes. What is unknown is how the intention to commitment occurs. There may be a variety of motives from intrinsic interest, to those influenced by rewards and status. There may be interest in playing squash by someone who wishes to keep fit, by someone who wishes to become for example a sports psychologist, or by someone who has enjoyed squash at home and wishes to find similar experiences at university.

The possibility that some people may find it difficult to become committed for a variety of personal reasons is important in the understanding of homesickness. The notion that psychoneurotic traits might predispose against commitment is supported by clinical observation and research. Loss of volition is typical of those suffering from depression; a possible strategic response to perceived high threat is a phobic response, namely, to withdraw and operate what Fisher (1984; 1986) termed 'control by avoidance'. A number of the homesick subjects studied were isolating themselves from the remainder of the students and appeared to stay in their rooms a great deal. Phobic response following the transition to university was found to be characteristic of the homesick (see Fisher & Hood, 1988).

However, we should not ignore the possibility that the features of the environment might directly encourage the operation of coping strategies which are passive or which have phobic characteristics. For example, a response pattern not unlike phobic avoidance might occur in situations of high demand as part of a 'shut down' strategy which excludes elements which are perceived as non-salient (see Miller, 1962). Thus, the sort of high-demand academic environment encountered at university might create response patterns which encourage homesickness.

A further development of the above notion is that the new environment does not just have a moderating role but has an active initiating role in creating and maintaining homesickness. This chapter explores some of the evidence which suggests that homesickness is a possible form of escapism in response to job strain. In fact as the research progressed it became apparent that university and college environments impose considerable strain on students. Although the patterns of strain change across the academic years for each student, the first year is one of the greatest periods of strain. Facing the pressures of academic and social demands seems to create job strain. Facing these pressures in the absence of direct parental support is an added factor; social support is in effect reduced just when it is needed.

It has previously been argued that post-transition environments are likely to be characterised by low control because the necessary knowledge and skills need to be evolved. Perception of low control creates a sense of helplessness or might in some cases be associated with raised effort and struggle for control. Either way, strain and distress are likely outcomes.

COGNITIVE APPRAISAL, COMMITMENT, AND ADAPTATION

One point that should be emphasised is that episodes of homesickness are apparently not confined to the first weeks following a move away from home. As part of the study reported by Fisher et al. (1985) involving university students, a group of second-, third-, and fourth-year students who remained in residence were investigated (Scottish universities have four-year degree courses). Comparison between first-years and post-first-years was difficult because they differed in age: the post-first-years were older (mean age = 19.6 years) as compared with the first-years (mean age = 18.6 years). However, age has not been found to be a factor in homesickness within the ranges studied.

Unexpectedly, the post-first-year group had homes which were less far away from the city of Dundee (in which the university is sited) than the first-year group. Therefore, remaining in residence may reflect complex factors such as the nearness of home.

Of the 25 post-first-years studied, 48% reported homesickness in the sixth week of the Autumn Term, although this was their second, third or fourth year at university. When asked to report the incidence of homesickness in the first year, the incidence level was 72%. A second, small, unpublished study involving 20 first-year students in the first-, second-, third- and fourth-year revealed homesick reporting levels of 68%, 50%, 48% and 10% respectively. Taken collectively, the studies indicate a progressive reduction of students reporting current feelings of homesickness with increasing duration of stay at university, but also emphasise that there are still some who feel homesick even after three academic years.

One factor of importance is that the homesick student is in a situation where his or her contact with home is re-established at roughly 10-week intervals. He or she is therefore constantly re-experiencing the break with home. Interestingly we found that for first-year students, the second term (after the Christmas break) showed a rise in the incidence of homesickness reporting (71–86%) and significantly greater frequency of homesickness reporting (average 4.4 on the scale from 0–5 as compared with an average of 3.2 in the first term). Certainly there was no evidence to indicate that the second break with home to attend university was less distressing in spite of the fact that by that time the student had had opportunity to make friends and establish a new life. Clearly, the break with home continues to have the capacity to be influential.

The adaptation process could be conceptualised in terms of the competing demands model on the assumption that with increasing time at university there is raised probability of commitment to some aspect of university life; sports, clubs, academic work, social life. These various sources of commitments increasingly replace home as a major source of rumination. The process of adaptation might therefore be strongly influenced by the kind of environment the new student discovers. If it is congenial and provides the kinds of facilities expected and required, adaptation will be favoured and homesickness reduced. Conversely hostile, unpleasant environments could be expected to have the opposite effects.

Commitment and satisfaction should depend crucially on the sort of appraisals a new student gives to the new environment as compared with the home environment. It follows that matching features of the new environment with the interests and orientation of the new student should facilitate adaptation. An environment which offers little in terms of interest should be more likely to reduce the liklihood of commitment and therefore should slow down or even prevent adaptation. One homesick student reported that in her normal home environment she was a regular church-goer and used to enjoy badminton with church groups in the local church hall. She could find badminton courts in the university environment but could not find a familiar church environment and could not find the special combination of badminton and church interest she was used to at home. This she said made her feel homesick—perhaps homesickness is therefore a response to an environment perceived as uncongenial or one in which the person recognises lack of satisfaction or lack of potential sources of commitment.

This fits with the findings that the homesick generally report less satisfaction with features of the new environment including the academic environment, features of residence, and social opportunities (see Fisher et al., 1985) and would be in keeping with the notion of congruence as proposed by Stokols, Schumaker and Martinez (1983) in accordance with which the mismatch between expectancies and reality create preconditions for adjustment difficulties.

This suggests the need to build a cognitive model in which appraisal of the qualities of the new environment as compared with the home environment are fundamental. Qualities of the new environment are assumed to be compared with the qualities of the home environment. At least initially, the university or college environment is likely to be lower in perceived security and higher in perceived challenge than the home environment. This was confirmed by asking a group of first-year students to rate in the first week of the first term on a five-category rating scale, some main features of the home and university environments. On a repeated measure statistic, the home environment was higher in security, comforts, and friendships, but lower in challenge, general demand, and in opportunities offered.

The appraisal of the degree to which loss of the comforts and securities can be offset by the challenge of the new environment could determine the likelihood of commitment to that new environment. However commitment may also be influenced by perceived demand levels and level of control afforded by the university or college environment.

SOURCES OF STRAIN IN EDUCATIONAL ENVIRONMENTS

Cognitive Appraisals of Home and College

Studies with university students have provided clues which suggest that the university environment is a source of strain, producing manifestations of distress in all students irrespective of whether or not they had left home to be newly residential, or remained home-based (see Fisher & Hood, 1987). This provides an important clue. Could it be that students when they first arrive at university, experience a severe form of stress at work? Could it be that homesickness in some students reflects this strain?

A further clue was reported in the above longitudinal study by Fisher and Hood (1987). As part of the study, students sampled in the sixth week of the first term were asked to indicate whether they were homesick 'currently' (on arrival at university) and whether they had been homesick 'initially' (at the time of assessment). Overall 71% reported being homesick either initially or currently or both; but of those who reported homesickness currently, 36.6% reported not having been homesick initially. In other words, homesickness appeared to have developed as the term progressed.

A further check on this involved examination of homesickness scores of 16 university students across the successive weeks of the term. Students were first asked to indicate on a five-point scale whether they were homesick in the sixth week of term. The 16 subjects who reported some level of homesickness then completed a serial profile (retrospective recall), beginning with the first week of arrival through to the (current) sixth week and then week by week until the tenth week of term. For nine subjects the trend was towards reduced homesickness reporting. This was significant on the Friedman Two-Way Analysis of Variance. For the remaining seven subjects the trend was from zero level initially towards increasing homesickness as the term progressed; there was a peak in the eighth week. Overall, the pattern of scoring was significant on the Friedman Two-Way Analysis of Variance. Comparisons between the first and last three weeks of term confirmed the above trends for each case.

The evidence suggesting that some subjects were not homesick initially but became so after some experience of the new university environment, suggests that homesickness might in some cases be a secondary response perhaps to perceived unpleasant aspects of the environment. One possibility is that the outcome of the appraisal of the security and comforts of home as compared with the discomfort and insecurity of the new environment (see previous sections in this chapter) leads to the perception of a mismatch in favour of the home environment. Perhaps then, home thoughts increasingly dominate cognition and may provide even an escape from confrontation with reality. In Chapter 7, it was proposed that the homesick subject might strategically increase the period of time engaged in thoughts of home as a response to a perceived adverse post-transition environment.

Demand and Control as Features of Work Strain Environments

The notion that some situations are associated with stress which is per-ceived as positive, whereas some situations are associated with negative stress, was noted by Selye (1974) who introduced the term 'eustress' to characterise positive stress environments. More recently, Karasek (1979) suggested that occupational environments which are stressful are best characterised by two variables—'demand' and 'low personal discretion (or control)'. When demand is high and discretion (or control) is high, the outcome is likely to be an experience which is positive and challenging. When demand is high but discretion or control is low, the outcome is more likely to be one of job strain and distress. Karasek developed this model following results from studies with Swedish and American workers in which those who reported job strain had jobs characterised by high demand and low discretion. In fact in many cases demand and control are likely to be interactive in that people with high control may use it to regulate or reduce demand. In spite of such difficulties, the principles of the job strain model do provide the possibility of obtaining some insights into the reasons for increase in homesickness as a function of time at university.

One possibility is that the student encountering a new university en-vironment experiences a period of job strain because demands are high and control is low because of the novelty of the new environment. (See control model outlined in Chapter 2.) The evidence that university creates a strainful environment was established in the context of a longitudinal study by Fisher and Hood (1987); all students, even those remaining in residence at home showed increased psychoneurotic symptoms following the transi-tion to university. Main reported problems were: 'academic demands' (reported by 65% of home-based and 61% of resident students); 'univer-sity routines and procedures' (reported by 35% of home-based and 24% of residents); social problems (reported by 24% of home-based students and 45% of residents); and financial (reported by 18% of home-based and 47% of resident students).

The possibility that features of the new environment may directly create homesickness is further supported by the results of studies involving both boarding school and university student populations, which were concerned with mobility history as a predictor of homesickness (Fisher et al., 1986; Fisher & Hood, 1988). It was found that homesickness was less likely in those who reported having been away from home for school or holidays but not for other reasons (such as summer jobs or staying with relatives). The selective nature of the self-reported mobility details might support the hypothesis proposing the operation of a self-selection factor; those who leave home for university and do not become homesick have also been willing to leave home for school or holiday residence in the past. Alternatively, it might be argued that certain experiences have an immunising effect in that individuals acquire resources if they learn to deal with the demands of new environments. Any finding which suggests that selective mobility experiences have an immunising effect on reaction to a current transition would provide indirect support for the job strain model: if leaving home *per se* is less critical than leaving home to experience an environment with properties in common with the current environment then clearly what is important is learning to cope with new institutional environments.

The job strain model would suggest that homesickness is a response to perceived high demands and low control. The possibility that job strain was caused by homesickness remains an alternative explanation. Two studies were carried out to investigate the hypothesis that perceived demand and perceived control levels differentiate the homesick from the non-homesick group.

Fifty-nine students took part in a study in which homesickness was assessed in the sixth week of the university term. Students provided written definitions of the term in the usual way and then indicated level of demand on a five-point scale from 'no demand' through to 'excessive demand'. They also indicated control on a five-point scale from 'no control' through to 'total control'. Both 'demand' and 'control' were defined for the subjects. 'Demand' was defined as the 'sum total of all threats and requirements imposed on a person'. 'Control' was defined broadly as 'the mastery and jurisdiction over all aspects of life at university'. As shown by Fig. 8.1, when the broad definition of control was provided, the 42 homesick subjects differed from their non-homesick counterparts in that they reported significantly higher demand ($p < 0.01$) but they did not differ in control levels. This does not support the job strain model.

One possible explanation for the result is that control was defined broadly as meaning all aspects of university life. Students typically have a great deal of control over their lives at university. They are treated for the most part as responsible adults although the system does have rules and sanctions. They can go home, miss days at the university, miss lectures etc. if they wish to. There are of course long-term penalties to be paid for this behaviour if it is persistent but at least the option remains. Therefore, it

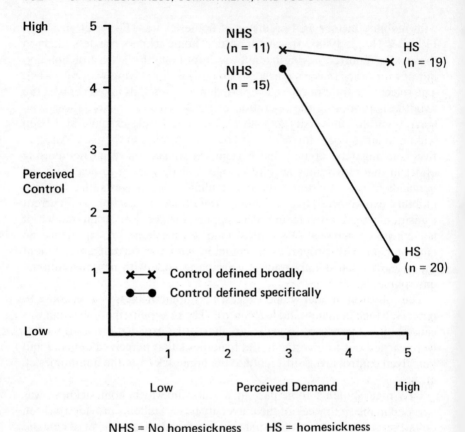

NHS = No homesickness   HS = homesickness

FIG. 8.1.   Perceived demand and control relationships for different definitions of control.

may be necessary to ask the question rather differently. The target for control arguably should be defined more specifically as 'control over the threats and requirements imposed by university life'.

A second study involving 35 new university students tested in the sixth week of the first university term, involved a specific definition of control. It was defined as 'power or mastery over acedamic work at university'. Otherwise the study remained the same as the previous study. The results showed that with a more specific definition of control the outcome was different. The homesick differed from the non-homesick both in terms of raised demand ($p < 0.01$) and lower control ($p < 0.001$). Thus the 'job strain' hypothesis, namely that homesickness may be a response to the distress created by the threats of the new environment receives some support.

One implication that researchers interested in the concept of control should note is that the way the concept is defined may have important implications for outcome. Fisher (1986) has argued that the concept is a broad umbrella term which encompasses mode for 'domain' and 'target' as identifiable qualifications. Control may be obtained by different modes; 'personal control' implies direct action on the situation; 'inter-personal control' implies action via inter-personal means. The latter may mean that a person pursues a goal by convincing another person (or persons) by argument or may try to achieve goals by disingenuous or manipulative techniques. Finally, an individual may operate via socio-political means to achieve a result.

In the case of target, the issue is even more complex. We need to ask the question 'control over what?' A person who apparently gives control over his aching tooth to a dentist, may do so because use of a skilled other is the most effective way of dealing with that particular problem. The target could be defined as 'to control the behaviour of the dentist' necessitates an inter-personal approach. Thus target can determine the domain of control.

Fisher (1987) has developed Epidemiological Problem Analysis as an approach to the investigation of stress in work environments. Each work environment is assumed to create potential problems for the individual. Having control over those problems means being able to reverse most of them and minimise their impact. Initial studies have shown that problems over which there is low control, persist longer and generate greater mental demands on the individual. Studies have also indicated that worry levels are greater in cases where there is perceived low control over problems. The data generally fit with the view that control is usually used to reduce demand. In other words the concepts are interactive.

For a student, becoming committed should mean that although demand is high there is an increasing chance of acquiring the personal and inter-personal skills which create the potential for operating control. Put quite simply, the committed student has the opportunity to acquire coping resources. Energy is directed towards finding out about how the organisation functions, what the rules and procedures are, what time meals are held or sporting fixtures and social events take place, how timetables are organised, where the venues for lectures are, etc. Becoming committed means that involvement creates new planning structures and 'expert knowledge' of how the system works. Thus the committed person has a greater potential for gaining control and reducing job strain; unless commitment creates new problems such as 'workaholic' patterns in those who become too committed and involved.

From what has been stated in previous chapters, the process of becoming committed may provide information sources which effectively compete for attentional resources and which attenuate homesickness. Commitment is envisaged as one of the major factors in the experience and continuation of homesickness. The post-transition environment and personality factors, such as depressed tendency, may alter the probability of commitment and hence change the likelihood of homesickness. Once homesickness is established then commitment becomes more difficult. It is likely that a positive feedback loop is established whereby a homesickness experience may be self-potentiating because of withdrawal and lack of commitment.

Putting together the two sets of ideas we can now see that the initial interactions the new student has with the environment may be crucial in determining experience of homesickness and subsequent adaptation. First, as established earlier in the book, if there is strong commitment, any adverse effects from the break in immediate contact with home can be ameliorated, whereas failure to become committed may create suitable conditions for homesickness experience. Secondly, universities provide strainful environments. For the student who perceives job strain, home may be increasingly favoured as the desirable alternative and this may create reveries or periods of mental escapism, as described in the second part of the previous chapter.

COGNITIVE APPRAISALS IN THE POST-TRANSITION ENVIRONMENT

It is hypothesised that following transition from home there is a period of cognitive appraisal of new circumstances relative to the home environment. The new environment offers more challenge and opportunity but probably less by way of comfort and security. As shown in Fig. 8.2, two sets of weightings may be involved: First there is the weighting of the qualities of the home environment as compared with the new environment. Secondly there is a weighting in terms of demand and control levels associated with the new environment. This is the computation which may determine whether or not the job strain is perceived. The individual who perceives low control over academic life will be likely to experience job strain. In such cases, the environment is no longer challenging but threatening and the response to this could be 'secondary' homesickness where reveries of the past predominate as a form of escapism or even as part of the decision making about returning home.

SUMMARY AND CONCLUSIONS

This chapter has been concerned with the role of the post-transition environment in the occurrence of homesickness. A distinction is made between the role of the new environment as a source of information which can compete with homesick thoughts created by the break with home, and

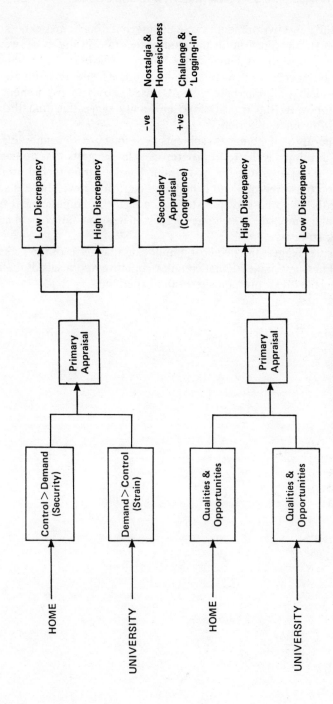

FIG. 8.2. A computational job strain model of homesickness.

the role of the new environment in actually precipitating homesickness as a result of job strain. Since in all the studies reported in this book we are dealing with transitions to demanding school and university environments there may be special circumstances. All students and student nurses, whether resident or home-based, show raised scores in psychoneurotic symptoms following the transition to university suggesting that the environment is a source of strain.

About one-third of homesick subjects are not homesick initially; the experience develops as the term progresses. This suggests that homesickness may be a response to perceived strain. The job strain model predicts that strain occurs when demand is high and control is low. There is some support for the hypothesis of job strain as a factor in homesickness from the results of a study which examines perceived demand and control levels in homesick students.

These results suggest the need for a multicausal analysis of the problem of homesickness and indicate that complex cognitive appraisals of the new environment may be a prerequisite of the experience.

9

A Multi-Causal Cognitive Theory of Homesick Experience

It is a daunting task to try to piece together the clues provided by the variety of main research findings on homesickness experience. Studies have been confined to the specific case of leaving home to reside in institutions for educational purposes and the data is incomplete leaving important gaps in our knowledge because it has been impossible to undertake all the studies desirable. In spite of this, there do seem to be some indications of the importance of the role of separation, loss, and interruption of life style, and factors in the post-transition environment.

In this chapter the aim is to take a risk and try to draw together some of the most important findings in order to begin to understand the processes involved in the distress associated with homesickness. Part of this chapter leads to the specification of a descriptive multi-causal or composite model which brings together most of the evidence reviewed in preceding chapters. A working model is proposed of how homesickness might be created in various contexts. Central to the model is the notion of an attentional resource which can be dominated by past plans and imagery. Once the attentional resource is determined by the past, insecurity is prepetuated because of the inappropriate thoughts which prevail. Also, the sense of loss is revitalised.

THE NATURE OF THE HOMESICKNESS EXPERIENCE

It has been established that homesickness is a complex state accompanied by past-centred ruminative activity. The psychological state has cognitive-emotional-motivational components and is often associated with distress.

It appears similar to grief and yet the individual knows that the previous environment continues to exist, and can be visited and even returned to on a permanent basis. In that sense the antecedents of homesickness are not comparable to bereavement and irreversible loss.

Any theory which explains the homesickness reaction must take account of main psychological features. There is attentional focus on ruminative activity concerned with home. In severe cases, the ruminative activity occurs compulsively. The homesick differ from their non-homesick counterparts who also focus on home but are more likely to be concerned with home problems or problems arising as a result of leaving home. This appears to be a qualitative difference between the homesick and their non-homesick counterparts. It is possible that the imagery for the homesick reflects differences in the sensitivity to the break with home, the intensity of the home experience, or reflects fundamental differences in planning processes.

Biological Models of Homesickness

A bilogical model would assume that ruminative activity which is home-centred is associated with distress and arises as an epiphenomenon due to the operation of biological mechanisms activated by loss and interruption. One way this could occur is if the absence of particular sets of neural signals activates alarm responses. Ruminative states then occur as a result of internal searches for expected and appropriate signals. In other words, this model would envisage loss as causing a sudden drop of control. Bowlby (1969) described the anxious searching of the infant who loses visual contact with the mother. It would be important that representations of the mother remain dominant in memory whilst searching continues; therefore imagery would dominate attention.

As described early in the book, a model which would provide a basis for understanding the effects of loss is the ideomotor model described by Greenwald (1970), based partly on the principle of reafference described by Von Holst (1954) (see Chapter 2). The model assumes that every command to the motor system evokes a neural copy. As illustrated in Fig. 2.1, the neural copy is assumed to have the capacity to evoke an expected signal from memory. In other words, the individual acts in relation to the world around him and the copy of each action can evoke an *expectancy* about what will happen as a result. This can then be used to compare with the *real* result of action. The resulting discrepancy generates alarm. (This is described in greater detail in Fisher, 1986, p. 75.) The codes available for predicting consequences from action are capable of describing and anticipating real events, and are assumed to evoke imagery which can provide a focus for consciousness.

Illustrating this example if it is assumed that the mother is a focus for attention in the infant, action systems will be organised around the mother-figure. The sudden disappearance of the mother's image means that actions designed to evoke expectancies of the mother-figure, no longer produce that effect. In terms of the ideomotor model, the neural copy of action comes to evoke expected consequences which do not occur in real life. Thus, an alarm process is set off and the infant engages in search behaviour in order to restore the reafferent signals that are expected.

The removal of a loved object could be assumed to produce neural mismatches creating the breakdown of stability resulting in searching behaviour and strong ruminative activity which directs searching. We could envisage such a biological account as providing an explanation of home-sickness as a response to leaving home. The fact that the individual *knows* that the loss is reversible would then be irrelevant because the neural systems are reacting to the absence of images.

Cognitive Accounts of Homesickness

The Persistence of Plans.   A cognitive model could account for home-sickness by assuming that persistence of thoughts and themes from the past is an intrinsic feature of cognitive adjustment to transitions, but creates distress whilst adjustment is happening. A planning process which capital-ises on the past in this way could be very adaptive in that resources and experiences can form the basis of new plans.

The view that plans are organised in ways that favour the persistence of past themes would imply a quantitative rather than a qualitative difference between homesick and non-homesick groups. Yet as shown in Chapter 7, there is evidence of a qualitative difference in the content of home-related ruminative activity in the homesick as compared with non-homesick counterparts. In the former case intrusive episodes from the past are domi-nant. In the latter case problems arising from the results of transition are prevalent.

Psychological Addiction.   An alternative approach which might pro-vide some basis for understanding the persistence of strong ruminative activity associated with transient or irreversible loss, is that the individual has become psychologically *addicted* to the security and comforts of aspects of the pre-transition environment. Home-related ruminations would be assumed to persist because they represent needs just like hunger or thirst. The studies have indicated that the homesick have very strong desires to go home. They miss the physical comforts and protections of home and use phrases such as 'my own room'; 'decent cooking'; 'being looked after'; 'a retreat from the world'.

The addiction model is given further support by the memory studies reported earlier which show that not only are thoughts of home dominant in the homesick but there is a valence factor operating, in that home is more rapidly associated with pleasant thoughts than with negative thoughts. The reverse is the case for the new university environment. This is consistent with the hypothesis that the homesick are psychologically addicted to home.

Congruence Between Actual and Desired Conditions. A cognitive approach which depends on appraisal and evaluation is that the new environment has qualities which are seen as undesirable or negative, in comparison with the home environment. This is supported by data from Fisher et al., 1985 and also by Kane, 1987 (see Chapter 5). The individual in the early stages of post-transition experience, perceives home as having superior and desired qualities. This creates a situation of *incongruence* where a person is continuing to exist in one environment whilst preferring to live in a different environment. In answer to the question 'why do you stay here (at university) if you are so homesick?', 57% of 85 students gave answers which suggest that giving up would upset parents/family; 14% thought it to be a sign of weakness; 21% thought of the implications for future career; the remainder indicated hope that the situation might improve.

Research on job strain has identified the importance of fit between the person and the environment (PE Fit) as a major factor (Van Harrison, 1978). Two kinds of fit have been identified. The first is the match between the skills and abilities of the individual and the demands of the job. The second is the extent to which the environment meets the individual's needs. A good person-environment fit occurs if the job factors are within the capabilities of the individual and when the total job environment meets the needs of the individual in terms of money, social facilities and opportunities for achievement.

Whilst university environments provide a student with opportunities for advancement, many other needs are not necessarily met. For example, 47% of university residents reported financial problems ranging from feelings of poverty to concern about management of limited resources; 45% of university residents reported problems of a social nature ranging from 'lack of privacy' to 'noise caused by other people'; 'being laughed at'; 'not finding any friends'; 'feeling ill at ease in an institution'; (see Fisher & Hood, 1987).

Van Harrison indicates that a poor person-environment fit at work is predictive of poor health and dissatisfaction. Raised symptom levels associated with poor fit include anxiety, complaints of insomnia, restlessness, increased smoking, over-eating, blood pressure, and serum cholesterol levels. However, the complex relationship between job features, satisfaction and mental health is not easily explained on the PE Fit model. For example there are cases of dissatisfaction at work but no changes in mental health. Workers may dislike, but nevertheless are not affected by, some conditions at work. In the case of homesick subjects both dissatisfaction and distress are involved and the PE Fit model might provide an account of the origins of unhappiness. Thus, congruence between desired and expected conditions determines the outcome.

Job Strain. The evidence collectively suggests that the university environment creates strain for students: Fisher and Hood (1987) provided evidence of increased distress following transition for residents and non-residents alike. Thus one viable possibility is that job strain created by the new environment is greater for some students and creates the pre-conditions for homesickness (see previous chapter). The individual who experiences job strain is assumed to be engaged in a cognitive appraisal in which home is seen as highly desirable, not necessarily because of the direct comforts offered (as outlined in the previous section above on congruence), but because home creates less demand and greater control; it is thus less challenging and more secure. The need to go home and the preoccupation with home is a logical outcome.

This view gains support from the finding that for some homesick students (perhaps about one-third) the experience increases as the term progresses. Also, as shown previously, 'demand' is perceived as high for all students but for the homesick students 'control', defined specifically as ability to influence aspects of the academic environment, is perceived of as low. If job strain creates homesickness then the domination of attention by thoughts of home is best seen as a form of escapism or may reflect decision-making concerning the return home.

THEORIES OF HOMESICKNESS AND THE ATTENTIONAL RESOURCE MODEL

The New Environment as Competing Demand

The accounts described in the previous section concern possible *reasons* for nostalgic content in the thoughts of the homesick. A second critical issue is, however, the dominance of home ruminations. Since the day's events appear able to keep these ruminations alternated for the majority of homesick subjects, a model is suggested in which the new environment provides information which competes for resources with homesick ruminations. Thus, as represented in Fig. 9.1, the features of the new environment provide the potential for the *attenuation* of homesick thoughts caused by

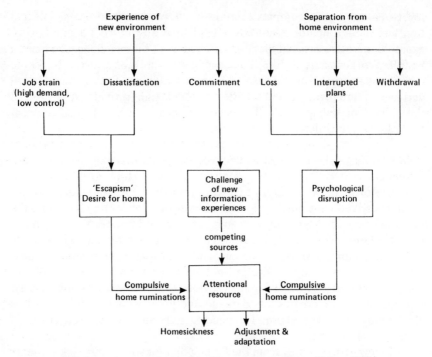

FIG. 9.1.   A composite model of homesickness. (From Fisher, 1988.)

leaving home. The greater the degree of commitment to the new environment, the greater the chance that there will be effective competing streams of information. Those depressed may lack the capacity to become committed and thus would be less likely to benefit from the potential sources of information provided by the new environment.

The New Environment as a Creator of Homesickness

An essentially different role could be envisaged for the new environment. As already described, perceived dissatisfaction with the new environment is greater for homesick students. In this case, the result of cognitive appraisals concerning the unpleasant features of the new environment as compared with the home environment, are fundamental.

Equally, circumstances of perceived job strain as computed by the individual (see Fig. 8.2), have been argued to create pre-conditions for homesickness. The individual may 'escape' by means of mental fantasies of happiness at home, or may continue to plan for visits home, thus creating the experience of continuous home thoughts. This process might be a form of 'hedonising', in that there are short-term pleasures associated with thoughts of home, but there may be long-term penalties in that the break with home is revitalised.

THE PRINCIPLES OF A MULTI-CAUSAL DESCRIPTIVE THEORY OF HOMESICKNESS: THE COMPOSITE MODEL

Of all the findings reported there are a number of key findings and it is useful to summarise them. Collectively, they suggest the need for a multi-causal model.

1. Homesickness is a complex syndrome in which preoccupation with the home and the past are paramount and associated with distress.
2. Homesickness appears to be largely independent of age factors or sex differences.
3. Episodes of homesickness are self-reported for about 50–70% of most populations studied when there is a prompted decision.
4. The episodes occur in the morning or at night suggesting that the day's activities have the capacity to keep homesickness at bay.
5. Episodes of homesickness thoughts are more likely during passive tasks and during 'mental' rather than physical activity.
6. Severely homesick individuals (about 10–15%) report the experience of homesickness to be continuous (non-episodic).
7. Homesickness subjects score higher on psychoneurotic symptoms and absent-mindedness as compared with their non-homesick counterparts. They have difficulties with concentration suggesting that control over the attentional mechanism is affected.
8. Homesick subjects are more likely to report low decisional control over the move, to be separated from home by greater physical distance and to be depressed prior to leaving home.
9. Homesick subjects are more likely to have intrusive trains of home-related thoughts rather than to be worrying about problems created by the move, or by problems which exist prior to the move.
10. Homesick subjects perceive home in positive terms and are fast to produce positive thoughts of home and negative thoughts of university.
11. The new university environment provides a source of strain for all students as evidenced by increases in psychoneurotic symptoms for resident and home-based students alike.
12. Homesick subjects are more likely to be dissatisfied with university and to report high demand and low control—the ingredients associated with job strain in other occupational settings.

13. Those who have left home to reside in an institution before, are less likely to report homesickness. Leaving home for other reasons may not ameliorate homesickness.

Figure 9.1 provides a descriptive, composite model of homesickness. Separation from home may operate via a number of psychological processes to cause a period of disruption and distress. The common denominators may be separation, interruption, loss of control, or change in role as the individual confronts his new world. But it is clear that ultimately we need to understand the persistence and domination of ruminative activity in directing attention.

Early in the book, the notion of competing demands on an attentional resource was introduced; it can be swamped or dominated by homesick ruminations. We have located relatively few personal factors which predict the occurrence of homesickness; circumstantial and situational factors seem more important. However, we have located depressed mood prior to leaving home as a predictor of subsequent homesickness. One explanation is that commitment to the new environment provides a rich source of new and challenging information which can compete effectively to attenuate home ruminations in the limited capacity attentional resource but the depressed are less likely to become committed to the new environment thus curbing its potential for attenuating homesickness.

Gilbert (1988) identifies the possibility that the depressed may, for good biological reasons, fail to become overtly committed to challenges. Dominance orders in the animal kingdom are preserved and winners protected from continual battles with revitalised losers, if loss of volition occurs. This would suggest that the depressed are unlikely to rise to tackle new challenges effectively and is supported by laboratory findings by Fisher (1986, Chapter 7).

Failure to become committed to the new environment may also occur if a person has expectancies which create incongruence. Poor residential features, difficult psychosocial environments, and lack of money may all contribute to a feeling of lack of well-being, which may delay or prevent commitment to the new environment. Thus, the effect of circumstantial as well as personal factors can be accomodated.

Although commitment is a vital component of the process of adjustment, it could be that very strong psychological disruption due to leaving home may effectively block it. Badly homesick students appear withdrawn and less likely to take part in the full range of university life. Lying in bed late in the mornings may be an indication of this. Thus there is the possibility that severe threat due to loss, separation, or interruption may itself create poor conditions for coping.

One of the possibilities not originally envisaged is that the new environment does not merely provide an aid to coping and adjustment to transition, but may actively *precipitate* homesickness. In particular, British boarding schools and universities are high pressure work environments with penalties for failure and rewards for success. The very complexity of a new institutional system may overwhelm students. Homesickness may develop as the student fails to gain control of the daily perceived demand. Seen in this way, homesickness might be an escape, a craving for security and lack of stress.

Escapism may take many forms but psychological escape into reveries of the pleasures of home-life, carries penalties because the distress of separation and loss are less likely to be perpetuated. The short-term gain of 'hedonising' is counterbalanced by the long-term consequences of perpetuating the homesickness experiences and lack of adaptation and adjustment. It could be considered to be a coping strategy with adverse consequences.

Figure 9.1 thus illustrates two roles for the new environment. First, it may be influential in *encouraging the commitment necessary to attenuate the dominance of home thoughts* in cognition. Equally the new environment, if perceived as strainful and unpleasant, may *create the pre-conditions for homesickness*. The conclusions from the studies strongly favour a multi-causal model in which the post-transition environment has major roles to play.

IMPLICATIONS FOR A THEORY OF PLANNING AND ATTENTION

One of the important considerations is that attention is (a) dominated by intrusive imagery from the past, or (b) is actively directed towards the past as either a means of escaping from the present environment, or (c) is an epiphenomenon which accompanies planning to go home.

The idea of internal and external sources of information competing for a limited capacity attentional resource is descriptive and provides little explanation of why home-orientated ruminations often have such compelling and uncontrollable characteristics. One critical question of interest is whether focus on home is mechanically determined by separation and interruption or whether it is strategic.

Understanding might be furthered by analogy with an hydraulic model in which needs create demands on available capacity in the attentional resource. This is in effect a loss of attentional control. Just as a drug addict thinks of the drug which is needed, or the hungry person thinks of food, so the homesick person thinks of home. A mechanism which creates pressure on attentional resources as a result of deprivation would be biologically advantageous. Need-related arousal might serve to direct energy towards solutions to the need. Attentional focus is mechanically determined in these circumstances. Mechanical control of attention by need-arousal can be overcome by effort to select other sources of information. Thus the committed person might overcome the demands created by need and is less likely to be homesick.

However, attention might be strategically as well as mechanically controlled. By actively deciding to think about home a person may escape mentally from the realities of the new environment. It might be assumed that active selection of sources of information, including home-related content, might be a powerful form of attentional control.

SUMMARY AND CONCLUSIONS

This chapter is concerned with drawing together some of the findings firstly in the form of a descriptive, multi-causal model of homesickness. The new (post-transition) environment is assumed to have two roles. First there is the possibility that it moderates the homesickness experience caused by loss, separation, interruption, loss of control or role change, because it provides competing sources of information.

Secondly, it might be responsible for creating homesickness in subjects, especially when it is not compatible with expectations or when there is perceived job strain.

Ultimately a working model is needed in which 'internal' self-focused thoughts compete with external sources of information in dominating resources. An hydraulic model of attention is proposed in which specific arousal mechanisms, once activated, raise the power of internal or external signals to dominate attentional resources. Active selection of home thoughts can occur if the need, and hence the associated arousal level, is great enough.

Circumstances or personal factors which encourage lack of commitment to the new environment raise the power of internal signals to dominate attention.

10 Helping the Homesick: An Attentional Management Approach

In this chapter, consideration is given to the issues of prevention and management. Those who deal with the residents of institutions are faced with the real problem of how to cope with those who are seriously distressed following the move from home. Those who are in care-giving or counselling roles in institutions may not always be in a position to become involved unless consulted directly, and as was indicated earlier in this book, there may be personal bias against reporting the experience of homesickness. Thus, the sorts of individuals who are actually seen by counsellors or doctors may be self-selected in that they admit to experiencing a problem or are forced by friends or wardens of residences to seek advice.

Studies reported in previous chapters have suggested that the signs of homesickness are likely to include depression, withdrawal, absent-mindedness, anxiety, and phobic avoidance accompanied by strong obsessive ruminative activity centred on home. There may be a number of presenting symptoms which have properties in common with agitated depression. The counsellor or doctor may need to make the diagnosis based both on context (newly moved from home) and the existence of compulsive ruminations focused on home. Homesickness may be seen as a specific manifestation of post-traumatic stress syndrome.

In the Appendix we have provided details of a diagnostic test which was designed to assess level of homesickness. It is possible to be distressed for a variety of reasons when experiencing a new educational institution. Home-based students may be distressed because they feel isolated and lost at university. Residents may be, in addition, affected by the break with home and are distinguished by the risk of homesickness.

THE EFFICACY OF STRESS-MANAGEMENT
PROGRAMMES

Generally, the distress and incompetence produced by traumatic experience of one kind or another is responsive to intervention. There is now substantial literature on the effectiveness of different forms of intervention, from changing the situation (attacking the problem directly) to helping the person see the situation differently and adjust to it. One of the greatest difficulties is in the setting up of rigorous criteria; any attention focused on a patient may lead to self-report of perceived improvement. There is great equivalence of outcome across different forms of treatment, which might suggest that a common mechanism is involved.

One possibility is that the common mechanism is that of self-esteem. A study of the interaction of intervention and self-esteem by de Paulo, Brown, Ishie, and Fisher (1981) showed that high self-esteem subjects performed better on a second task if they had been given helpful information on their performance (contrived to be low) on a first task, whereas the reverse was true for low self-esteem subjects.

Similarly Loeb, Beck, and Diggory (1971) showed that the depressed are more likely to react adversely to negative feedback than the non-depressed. The latter show improvements on a second task if provided with evidence suggesting failure on a first task. The former only responded positively to success and encouragement.

Taken collectively, therapists and counsellors should be encouraged to respond to the distressed student by some preliminary assessment of personality factors such as self-esteem. Those who are strongly self-blaming with low self-esteem might need more concerted effort to achieve a positive result.

If, as seems to be true from the Fisher and Hood (1987) results, the mildly depressed are more likely to react adversely to transition, one preventative approach might be to target counselling resources on these individuals and to try to provide maximum encouragement to them to become committed.

Expression and Acknowledgement of Grief

Homesickness might well be viewed by non-sufferers and sufferers alike as a form of failure, weakness, or 'wimpishness'. As demonstrated in earlier parts of the book, whereas the response to bereavement is socially acceptable, the response to homesickness is not. Therefore, the very nature of the experience, its social sanctions and the reporting of it, might be associated with low self-esteem.

Irrespective of the cause of distress, its expression is important. In the case of bereavement, those unable to express grief and emotion are prone to later pathological reactions (see Parkes, 1972). Cultural climates created to encourage the expression of grief in public, fostered by some Middle and Far Eastern countries, are beneficial. The social unacceptability of homesickness means that the grief is likely to be confined to private moments as the *cause* of the emotion may be personally regarded as unacceptable or trivial. Part of the management of the experience might be to persuade the sufferer that the experience itself is a common one, that 60–70% of victims experience it, and that it is likely to diminish in intensity.

The distinction between problem-focused coping and emotion-focused coping (see Lazarus & Folkman, 1984) provides a useful distinction in many life and work stress environments. Problem-focused approaches are concerned with the cause of the stress. Thus a person facing a stressful problem might identify it as being due to the difficulties of meeting deadlines or of being passed over for promotion. It might then be possible to identify strategies for coping. Even so, Schönpflug and Batman (1988) warn of the dangers of adverse effects of coping strategies. A strategy designed to ameliorate a particular stressful problem may create other problems in the process. Seen in this light, even a confiding relationship, believed strongly to reduce the risk of depression as an outcome of social stress (see Brown and Harris, 1978) may have adverse consequences (revelation of a personal difficulty to someone else; the difficulty of not wanting to follow directives provided by the confident, and so on).

Problem-focused Coping

In the case of homesickness, the 'problem' is partly the conflict between the distress of leaving home and the pressure (or personal need) to remain in the new environment to fulfil an ambition to succeed in the world. Thus homesickness is a self-created condition in the way that bereavement is not. The homesick person could cure the existing problems by simply returning home. The cost might be the loss of opportunity for advancement, disappointed parents, or personal feelings of failure. One possibility is to compromise, return home, and continue with the same or a related form of training elsewhere.

Some students might be able to do this; nursing students particularly may find training in hospitals closer to home. Evidence during the research studies indicated that a higher incidence of giving up and returning home occurred in student nurses than in students at university. There may have been a number of reasons, but at least one is that a long-term career penalty may be less likely for student nurses. University students are more likely to be faced with a dilemma due to lack of alternative places; one medical student who was very distressed at Dundee, wrote to every medical school and university in the location of home to see if she could obtain a place. This behaviour sustains the conflict, because return home could have a damaging effect on future career prospects.

The problem for the homesick is therefore the conflict between a commitment to stay and a desire to go home. The problem-focused approach would mean re-evaluation of the original decision to leave home for educational/vocational advancement. If distress and general unhappiness is very great, this is what counsellors or those in care-taking roles might have to consider.

Attentional Manipulations

Findings reported in previous chapters suggest that for some homesick subjects the day's events may keep homesickness at bay, whereas for others the homesick experience is continuous. One suggestion, expressed in the form of a conceptual model—'the competing resource model'—is that commitment to the new (post-transition) environment helps to attenuate homesickness; it is assumed that the information generated by the new environment competes effectively for a limited capacity resource.

The implication for the management of homesickness is that involvement with the new environment, creates the potential for attenuation of the homesickness experience. There are two possibilities: one is to create the conditions for commitment; the other is to enforce commitment by use of rules and regulations which minimise periods of lack of involvement. The latter technique may be particularly useful in schools where new pupils can be kept busy by fixed activities, regularly prescribed. The activities should be physical rather than mental (sports, games, walks, trips to museums, etc.) and active rather than passive. The day of a school pupil cannot be dominated by these kinds of activities because the main purpose of the school is to create and encourage learning and scholarship. However, periods at the beginning of the term, during the early and late part of the day and at weekends, could be directed in ways which will keep pupils busy and if possible physically active.

In the case of groups who have more control over their life activities, it may be necessary to train individuals to create commitment. This could be further targetted in that those who report homesickness can be detected prior to leaving home by raised levels of depression (Fisher & Hood, 1987). This might indicate that there is a lack of commitment to the new environment (Fisher 1986, Chapter 7), and therefore lack of competing information which can effectively attenuate the ruminations caused by loss of home and by competition for the attentional resource.

The problem of encouraging commitment is that the individual concerned must participate and create the motivation. Whereas traditional theories have assumed that the depressed lack the volition for commitment (see Fisher, 1986). Kuhl and Kazen-Saad (1988) suggest that the depressed are perfectionists and become over-committed to a task. The difference in emphasis in relation to homesickness seems to be that on the first analysis it would be argued that depression indicates lack of ability to become committed to any environment/task. By contrast Kuhl's analysis would suggest that depression involves strong commitment to the previous environment. Therefore on the traditional analysis the depressed are assumed to fail to make use of the new environment for attenuating homesickness, whereas the non-depressed become committed and benefit accordingly. On the Kuhl model, the commitment to home should create the preconditions for homesickness (greater distress because of greater home dependency and involvement) and might also create lack of ability to utilise sources of interest in the new environment for attenuating homesickness. Thus, the Kuhl analysis makes provision for two variables in homesickness, whereas the traditional analysis makes provision for only one.

On either analysis, encouraging commitment would be an important management principle. This may have paradoxical elements because features associated with the homesickness reaction are withdrawal and depression. However, individuals can be persuaded to produce behaviour which they do not necessarily like. The counsellor should instruct the sufferer to increase the proportion of time spent in physical activity and to take up interests and hobbies. The latter course of action might be encouraged by the provision of facilities which match with interests in the home environment. Students might be encouraged to indicate their hobbies, sports, and interests in order of priority so that information about facilities could be provided and, where necessary, active encouragement to take up a high preference hobby could be given.

Instructions about the importance of increasing level of commitment could be given to the homesick students in order to create efforts in that direction. An added possibility is to direct actively the person by encouraged completion of a schedule. He or she could be instructed to create leisure periods during the week and to fill these leisure periods with desired activities of specified kinds decided in consultation with the counsellor concerned. An indirect spin-off will be the increased likelihood of social interactions which help to ward off loneliness and provide confiding relationships.

It is perhaps significant that Stokols et al. (1983) note the vulnerability of those individuals with 'low exploratory tendency' in new environments following transition. 'Low exploratory tendency' might represent lack of intended commitment to a new environment and may, therefore, increase the possibility of negative effects of transition.

SUMMARY AND CONCLUSIONS

Counselling and intervention for the homesick should involve some attempt to assess the self-esteem of the client and to try to rationalise and normalise the experience. A problem-orientated approach might be to quote the facts which suggest that at least a half to three-quarters of most people who leave home are likely to experience homesickness for a while.

If the distress reaction is serious, the conflict between remaining in the current place and returning home could be explored to see how great the sufferer's commitment is and especially to see if there are any alternative forms of education or training which could be home-based. The main approach however should be focused towards persuading sufferers to be committed to some aspects of the new environment. This includes participating in social and leisure activities. Any sporting interests should be encouraged. The ruminations which drive homesickness may be attenuated by the presence of competing information and this will in turn help to relieve distress and drive the adaptation process. The formation of self-help groups may provide simultaneously solutions to many of the main problems.

Attentional management therapy is strongly recommended as a fundamental method of dealing with the adverse effects of transition and loss. If intrusive competing sources of external information can be created the punishing ruminations of the homesick might be effectively attenuated. Thus, a practical management technique is indicated and progress in terms of adaptability should be assessed.

Appendix
The Dundee Relocation
Inventory: A Diagnostic Test
for the Assessment of
Homesickness and Distress
Following Transition

Throughout the book, homesickness has been self-assessed and it was established that although the written definitions of homesickness vary in length and have indiosyncratic components, homesick and non-homesick subjects do not appear to differ either in the number of component phrase-elements provided, or in the dominance order of features provided as indicated by report frequency. Thus all subjects indicate that preoccupation with home is paramount. Key features which create preoccupation and emotional response concern family, friends, home objects, and routines. Symptoms such as depression, unhappiness, grief, loss of appetite, dizziness, insomnia, and health-related fears, feature at subordinate levels in the definitions provided by subjects and appear to be highly varied and idiosyncratic. Attitudes to the new environment and its consequences are also included; these include negative appraisals of the new environment such as dislike of specified features, experience of being lost, overwhelmed, lonely, or afraid.

In all studies reported so far, the main form of measurement used has been the frequency measure of self-assessed homesickness. From this, a basic binary measure (homesick or non-homesick) can be obtained by dichotomising the scores into zero frequency and greater than zero frequency. In the retrospective student study (Fisher et al., 1985), the frequency measure was obtained from recall by students of the first five

---

NOTE: Keith Murray was responsible for the development of the early stages of the inventory and I am indebted to him for the initiatives and work involved. (Test copyright: Dr. S. Fisher and Mr. K. Murray.)

weeks of term. In the boarding school diary studies, the measure was calculated from the recalled daily episodes recorded across two weeks (Fisher et al., 1986).

The frequency measure is more satisfactory than the binary measure alone because it can distribute homesickness scores so that a range of response levels from zero to n can be obtained. There is a good case for developing a measure which enables homesickness to be assessed on the basis of answers to a specified number of prompted questions. Most depression inventories do not, for example, ask a person to define 'depression' and then assess depression frequency levels across a period of time; they involve scoring the responses to a number of different questions assumed to be assessing depression. This method involves the assumption that the positive endorsement of more attributes or symptoms means greater intensity level; i.e. a highly depressed person will provide positive endorsements on most items of the scale. This assumption is consistent with an hierarchial model of mental disturbance where more severity implies more symptoms and is implicit in most clinical questionnnaires.

THE CONSTRUCTION OF THE INVENTORY

The construction of the inventory involved three stages; item generation, item analysis and selection; item validation.

Item Generation

The initial stage consisted of generating a large number of items for potential later use in the inventory. The range had to be sufficiently great so as to ensure that no important items were omitted. The majority of the items were selected from the definitions provided by university students and boarding school pupils during ongoing studies (all of which have been described in earlier chapters). These were further augmented by other items which the research group considered to be likely to be appropriate.

Items were phrased in the form of statements and rated by subjects on an associated scale. Since rating scales were worded differently for different items, the questionnaires were divided into four groups, based on the different rating scales used. The four different scales are shown in Questionnaires A, B, C, and D. The first two questionnaires contained items with which the respondent indicated agreement; the third questionnaire involved intensity scales; the fourth questionnaire involved the intensity and frequency elements. The four questionnaires were randomised and completed by 326 first-year students randomly selected from populations at the universities of Edinburgh and Aberdeen. Testing occurred in the fifth and sixth weeks of the first term.

Each subject was asked to complete the questionnaire by endorsing the statement which best represented his or her current state. Completed questionnaires were returned anonymously to the Psychology Department at the University of Dundee in pre-stamped addressed envelopes. The completion rate was 79%.

Item Analysis

The subjects' response patterns were factor analysed. Both oblique and orthogonal factor solutions were obtained. The four orthogonal factors required 15 iterations and accounted for 66% of the cumulative variance.

The first factor which accounted for 45% of the variance was interpreted as being a *general adaptation* factor. Items loading on this factor were: 'I feel disorientated here'; 'I feel insecure here'; 'I feel threatened here'; 'I feel unsettled here'; 'I feel unable to cope here'; 'I feel unhappy here'; 'I feel uneasy here'; 'I feel unloved here'.

The second factor which accounted for 9% of the variance is christened *home factor*; items loading included: 'I miss my family'; 'I want to go home'; 'I would like to live further from my family'; 'When I have problems I contact my family'; 'I would like to go home more often than I do'; 'I cannot stop thinking about home'; 'When I visit home I find it hard to return here'; 'I think that home is better than here'; 'I wake up wishing I were at home';

The third factor accounting for 7% of the variance was christened *satisfaction factor*; items loading included: 'I feel very satisfied here'; 'I feel optimistic here'; 'I feel fulfilled here'; 'I feel excited about the work here'; 'I do not regret having moved here'; 'I made a mistake moving here';

The fourth factor accounting for 5% of the variance was christened *social factor*. Items loading were: 'I miss having someone close to talk to'; 'I feel needed here'; 'There are people in whom I can confide'.

The final form of the inventory involved selecting from the items which loaded on the four factors—with consideration for balance of pleasant-orientated items (e.g. 'I feel loved here'), and unpleasant items ('I feel unhappy here').

QUESTIONNAIRE A

Instructions

We are interested in finding out some things about you. Read each of the following statements and circle the statement which best describes your thoughts since having moved here.

Do not think too long about the meaning of any item. Be sure that you answer every question.

1. I feel unable to cope with novel situations.

| Disagree Strongly | Disagree Mildly | Unsure | Agree Mildly | Agree Strongly |

2. I am primarily responsible for my own actions.

| Disagree Strongly | Disagree Mildly | Unsure | Agree Mildly | Agree Strongly |

3. I would like to live further from my family.

| Disagree Strongly | Disagree Mildly | Unsure | Agree Mildly | Agree Strongly |

4. When I have problems I contact my family.

| Disagree Strongly | Disagree Mildly | Unsure | Agree Mildly | Agree Strongly |

5. I find it easy to make friends.

| Disagree Strongly | Disagree Mildly | Unsure | Agree Mildly | Agree Strongly |

6. I like travelling long distances by myself.

| Disagree Strongly | Disagree Mildly | Unsure | Agree Mildly | Agree Strongly |

7. I like to know what awaits me at the end of a journey.

| Disagree Strongly | Disagree Mildly | Unsure | Agree Mildly | Agree Strongly |

8. I would live anywhere for a good job.

| Disagree Strongly | Disagree Mildly | Unsure | Agree Mildly | Agree Strongly |

9. I would quite happily live in one place for life.

| Disagree Strongly | Disagree Mildly | Unsure | Agree Mildly | Agree Strongly |

Questionnaire A (continued)

10. When I leave home I feel lonely and insecure.

Disagree Strongly	Disagree Mildly	Unsure	Agree Mildly	Agree Strongly

11. I feel agitated on leaving home, even to go on holiday.

Disagree Strongly	Disagree Mildly	Unsure	Agree Mildly	Agree Strongly

12. I find home stressful.

Disagree Strongly	Disagree Mildly	Unsure	Agree Mildly	Agree Strongly

13. I like having to be self-reliant.

Disagree Strongly	Disagree Mildly	Unsure	Agree Mildly	Agree Strongly

QUESTIONNAIRE B

Instructions

Read each of the following statements and circle the statement which best describes your thoughts since having moved here.

Do not think for too long about the meaning of any item. Be sure that you answer every question.

1. I do not regret having moved here.

   | Disagree Strongly | Disagree Mildly | Unsure | Agree Mildly | Agree Strongly |

2. I made a mistake moving here.

   | Disagree Strongly | Disagree Mildly | Unsure | Agree Mildly | Agree Strongly |

3. I made a mistake moving from home.

   | Disagree Strongly | Disagree Mildly | Unsure | Agree Mildly | Agree Strongly |

4. My life has changed for the better since moving here.

   | Disagree Strongly | Disagree Mildly | Unsure | Agree Mildly | Agree Strongly |

5. I feel unable to improve my life here.

   | Disagree Strongly | Disagree Mildly | Unsure | Agree Mildly | Agree Strongly |

6. I would like to go home more often than I do.

   | Disagree Strongly | Disagree Mildly | Unsure | Agree Mildly | Agree Strongly |

7. I am satisfied with my present residence.

   | Disagree Strongly | Disagree Mildly | Unsure | Agree Mildly | Agree Strongly |

8. I hope to have more friends in the future than I have now.

   | Disagree Strongly | Disagree Mildly | Unsure | Agree Mildly | Agree Strongly |

9. I find myself making more errors and mistakes than normal.

   | Disagree Strongly | Disagree Mildly | Unsure | Agree Mildly | Agree Strongly |

10. I felt obliged to come here.

    | Disagree Strongly | Disagree Mildly | Unsure | Agree Mildly | Agree Strongly |

Questionnaire B (continued)

11. There are people here in whom I can confide.

| Disagree Strongly | Disagree Mildly | Unsure | Agree Mildly | Agree Strongly |

12. I have better friends here than I have at home.

| Disagree Strongly | Disagree Mildly | Unsure | Agree Mildly | Agree Strongly |

13. I cry less often than I did at home.

| Disagree Strongly | Disagree Mildly | Unsure | Agree Mildly | Agree Strongly |

14. I have lost my appetite lately.

| Disagree Strongly | Disagree Mildly | Unsure | Agree Mildly | Agree Strongly |

15. I feel cut off from the world here.

| Disagree Strongly | Disagree Mildly | Unsure | Agree Mildly | Agree Strongly |

16. I cannot stop thinking of home.

| Disagree Strongly | Disagree Mildly | Unsure | Agree Mildly | Agree Strongly |

17. I feel upset and lonely when I think of home.

| Disagree Strongly | Disagree Mildly | Unsure | Agree Mildly | Agree Strongly |

18. I think of past events here.

| Disagree Strongly | Disagree Mildly | Unsure | Agree Mildly | Agree Strongly |

19. When I visit home, I find it hard to return here.

| Disagree Strongly | Disagree Mildly | Unsure | Agree Mildly | Agree Strongly |

20. I feel that I belong here.

| Disagree Strongly | Disagree Mildly | Unsure | Agree Mildly | Agree Strongly |

21. I have many friends here.

| Disagree Strongly | Disagree Mildly | Unsure | Agree Mildly | Agree Strongly |

22. I think home is better than here.

| Disagree Strongly | Disagree Mildly | Unsure | Agree Mildly | Agree Strongly |

QUESTIONNAIRE C

Instructions

Read each of the following statements and judge how intensely you have felt this since moving here.

Do not think for too long about the meaning of any item. Be sure that you answer every question.

1. I miss home.

Never Felt	Very Mildly	Quite Mildly	Quite Strongly	Very Strongly

2. I dislike being here.

Never Felt	Very Mildly	Quite Mildly	Quite Strongly	Very Strongly

3. I feel disorientated here.

Never Felt	Very Mildly	Quite Mildly	Quite Strongly	Very Strongly

4. I feel unsettled here.

Never Felt	Very Mildly	Quite Mildly	Quite Strongly	Very Strongly

5. I miss my family.

Never Felt	Very Mildly	Quite Mildly	Quite Strongly	Very Strongly

6. I feel lonely here.

Never Felt	Very Mildly	Quite Mildly	Quite Strongly	Very Strongly

7. I feel unhappy here.

Never Felt	Very Mildly	Quite Mildly	Quite Strongly	Very Strongly

8. I feel insecure here.

Never Felt	Very Mildly	Quite Mildly	Quite Strongly	Very Strongly

9. I miss friends I have at home.

Never Felt	Very Mildly	Quite Mildly	Quite Strongly	Very Strongly

Questionnaire C (continued)

10. I want to go home.

| Never Felt | Very Mildly | Quite Mildly | Quite Strongly | Very Strongly |

11. I feel threatened here.

| Never Felt | Very Mildly | Quite Mildly | Quite Strongly | Very Strongly |

12. I miss having someone close to talk to.

| Never Felt | Very Mildly | Quite Mildly | Quite Strongly | Very Strongly |

13. I feel unloved here.

| Never Felt | Very Mildly | Quite Mildly | Quite Strongly | Very Strongly |

14. I feel uneasy here.

| Never Felt | Very Mildly | Quite Mildly | Quite Strongly | Very Strongly |

15. I feel unfamiliar here.

| Never Felt | Very Mildly | Quite Mildly | Quite Strongly | Very Strongly |

QUESTIONNAIRE D

Instructions

We are interested in finding out some things about you. Read each of the following statements and judge how often you have felt like this since having moved here. At the same time judge for how long this feeling lasts, on average. Indicate both these judgements by circling statements on the scales provided. Be sure that you answer every question.

1. I feel unable to cope here.

		(Frequency)		
Never	Rarely	Sometimes	Often	Always

		(Duration)		
Never	For Seconds	For Minutes	For Hours	For Days

2. I feel very satisfied here.

		(Frequency)		
Never	Rarely	Sometimes	Often	Always

		(Duration)		
Never	For Seconds	For Minutes	For Hours	For Days

3. I hate being here.

		(Frequency)		
Never	Rarely	Sometimes	Often	Always

		(Duration)		
Never	For Seconds	For Minutes	For Hours	For Days

4. I feel disorientated here.

		(Frequency)		
Never	Rarely	Sometimes	Often	Always

		(Duration)		
Never	For Seconds	For Minutes	For Hours	For Days

5. I feel unsettled here.

		(Frequency)		
Never	Rarely	Sometimes	Often	Always

		(Duration)		
Never	For Seconds	For Minutes	For Hours	For Days

Questionnaire D (continued)

6. I feel optimistic about life here.

		(Frequency)		
Never	Rarely	Sometimes	Often	Always

		(Duration)		
Never	For Seconds	For Minutes	For Hours	For Days

7. I wake up wishing that I were at home.

		(Frequency)		
Never	Rarely	Sometimes	Often	Always

		(Duration)		
Never	For Seconds	For Minutes	For Hours	For Days

8. I miss my family.

		(Frequency)		
Never	Rarely	Sometimes	Often	Always

		(Duration)		
Never	For Seconds	For Minutes	For Hours	For Days

9. I feel lonely here.

		(Frequency)		
Never	Rarely	Sometimes	Often	Always

		(Duration)		
Never	For Seconds	For Minutes	For Hours	For Days

10. I feel excited about work here.

		(Frequency)		
Never	Rarely	Sometimes	Often	Always

		(Duration)		
Never	For Seconds	For Minutes	For Hours	For Days

11. I feel unhappy here.

		(Frequency)		
Never	Rarely	Sometimes	Often	Always

		(Duration)		
Never	For Seconds	For Minutes	For Hours	For Days

Questionnaire D (continued)

12. I feel insecure here.

		(Frequency)		
Never	Rarely	Sometimes	Often	Always

		(Duration)		
Never	For Seconds	For Minutes	For Hours	For Days

13. I feel fulfilled here.

		(Frequency)		
Never	Rarely	Sometimes	Often	Always

		(Duration)		
Never	For Seconds	For Minutes	For Hours	For Days

14. I miss friends I have at home.

		(Frequency)		
Never	Rarely	Sometimes	Often	Always

		(Duration)		
Never	For Seconds	For Minutes	For Hours	For Days

15. I want to go home.

		(Frequency)		
Never	Rarely	Sometimes	Often	Always

		(Duration)		
Never	For Seconds	For Minutes	For Hours	For Days

16. I feel confident here.

		(Frequency)		
Never	Rarely	Sometimes	Often	Always

		(Duration)		
Never	For Seconds	For Minutes	For Hours	For Days

17. I feel isolated from the world.

		(Frequency)		
Never	Rarely	Sometimes	Often	Always

		(Duration)		
Never	For Seconds	For Minutes	For Hours	For Days

Questionnaire D (continued)

18. I think of past events.

		(Frequency)		
Never	Rarely	Sometimes	Often	Always
		(Duration)		
Never	For Seconds	For Minutes	For Hours	For Days

19. I feel threatened here.

		(Frequency)		
Never	Rarely	Sometimes	Often	Always
		(Duration)		
Never	For Seconds	For Minutes	For Hours	For Days

20. I miss having someone close to talk to.

		(Frequency)		
Never	Rarely	Sometimes	Often	Always
		(Duration)		
Never	For Seconds	For Minutes	For Hours	For Days

21. I feel unloved here.

		(Frequency)		
Never	Rarely	Sometimes	Often	Always
		(Duration)		
Never	For Seconds	For Minutes	For Hours	For Days

22. I feel needed here.

		(Frequency)		
Never	Rarely	Sometimes	Often	Always
		(Duration)		
Never	For Seconds	For Minutes	For Hours	For Days

23. I feel uneasy here.

		(Frequency)		
Never	Rarely	Sometimes	Often	Always
		(Duration)		
Never	For Seconds	For Minutes	For Hours	For Days

Questionnaire D (continued)

24. I feel unfamiliar here.

		(Frequency)		
Never	Rarely	Sometimes	Often	Always

		(Duration)		
Never	For Seconds	For Minutes	For Hours	For Days

25. I miss home.

		(Frequency)		
Never	Rarely	Sometimes	Often	Always

		(Duration)		
Never	For Seconds	For Minutes	For Hours	For Days

FIRST VERSION OF THE DUNDEE RELOCATION
INVENTORY

The first version of the Dundee Relocation Inventory is illustrated in Questionnaire E. The questionnaire was designed using binary responses to each of 26 questions including two dummy questions: 'I forget people's names'; and 'When I do a job I do it well'. The subjects wer 34 home-based first-year students and 64 first-year residents. Analysis of the results showed that home-based students were not discriminated from residents, but that the homesick residents were discriminated from the non-homesick residents on the following items: 'I miss home' ($p < 0.001$); 'I feel optimistic about life here' ($p < 0.01$); 'I miss having someone close to talk to' ($p < 0.05$); 'I miss my family' ($p < 0.001$); 'I would like to go home more often than I do' ($p < 0.01$); 'I feel lonely here' ($p < 0.01$). The mean DRI score for non-homesick residents was 4.0 (S.D. = 3.2) and the mean score for homesick residents was 8.5 (S.D. = 4.2). The difference was statistically significant: $p < 0.001$ (see Fisher & Hood, 1987).

QUESTIONNAIRE E
FIRST VERSION—DUNDEE RELOCATION INVENTORY

Instructions

Read each of the following statements carefully and circle the YES or NO opposite each, depending upon which one best fits how you have felt recently. Do not think for too long about any one statement and be sure to circle either YES or NO for each one.

I forget people's names.	YES	NO
When I do a job I do it well.	YES	NO
I feel able to cope here.	YES	NO
I miss home.	YES	NO
I feel optimistic about life here.	YES	NO
I miss having someone close to talk to.	YES	NO
I feel happy here.	YES	NO
I miss my family.	YES	NO
I feel fulfilled here.	YES	NO
I feel unloved here.	YES	NO
I feel unsettled here.	YES	NO

Questionnaire E (continued)		
When I have problems I contact my family.	YES	NO
I feel excited about work here.	YES	NO
I feel needed here.	YES	NO
I feel uneasy here.	YES	NO
I would like to go home more often than I do.	YES	NO
I regret having moved here.	YES	NO
There are people here in whom I can confide.	YES	NO
I feel secure here.	YES	NO
I cannot stop thinking of home.	YES	NO
I feel very satisfied here.	YES	NO
I have many friends here.	YES	NO
I wake up wishing that I were home.	YES	NO
I made a mistake moving here.	YES	NO
I feel lonely here.	YES	NO

SECOND VERSION OF THE DUNDEE RELOCATION INVENTORY

It was clear from the previous results that the discriminatory items for homesickness focused on the questions concerned with missing home. Distress and disorientation can affect all students in a new environment; transitions which do not involve a change of residence can also be stressful (see Brown and Armstrong, 1986; Fisher & Hood, 1987). It makes sense to find that really it is only the antecedent conditions represented in cognition that provide the important means for discrimination. This raises an interesting issue; states of mental disturbance should perhaps be classified in terms of the associated cognitions rather then the symptoms which result. Thus distress which results from loss and where loss-cognitions are dominant, would be discriminably different from distress resulting from, for example, failure. The fact that the form of the distress might vary would be considered in terms of the central cognitive themes. Thus the early stages of reversible loss could be associated with raised anxiety and distress whereas failure and irreversible loss might be associated with apathy, loss of volition and helplessness.

The second version of the DRI is provided in Questionnaire F. It involved the introduction of a three-category rating scale; the subject scored from zero to two on each of the questions. The scoring was reversed for negative items. Thus the counterbalance of negative and positive statements was not sacrificed in order to introduce the rating scale. Introduction of the three-category scale had the effect of driving apart the scores of the homesick and non-homesick. For a sample of 34 non-homesick students the mean score was 5.3 (S.D. = 1.1) whereas for a sample of 51 homesick subjects the mean score was 17.5 (S.D. = 3.9). The difference was significant ($p < 0.001$).

QUESTIONNAIRE F
SECOND VERSION—DUNDEE RELOCATION INVENTORY

I forget people's names.	Never	Sometimes	Often
When I do a job I do it well.	Never	Sometimes	Often
I feel able to cope here.	Never	Sometimes	Often
I miss home.	Never	Sometimes	Often
I feel optimistic about life here.	Never	Sometimes	Often
I miss having someone close to talk to.	Never	Sometimes	Often
I feel happy here.	Never	Sometimes	Often
I miss my family.	Never	Sometimes	Often
I feel fulfilled here.	Never	Sometimes	Often
I feel unloved here.	Never	Sometimes	Often
I feel unsettled here.	Never	Sometimes	Often
When I have problems I contact my family.	Never	Sometimes	Often
I feel excited about work here.	Never	Sometimes	Often
I feel needed here.	Never	Sometimes	Often
I feel uneasy here.	Never	Sometimes	Often
I would like to go home more often than I do.	Never	Sometimes	Often
I regret having moved here.	Never	Sometimes	Often
There are people here in whom I can confide.	Never	Sometimes	Often
I feel secure here.	Never	Sometimes	Often
I cannot stop thinking of home.	Never	Sometimes	Often
I feel very satisfied here.	Never	Sometimes	Often
I have many friends here.	Never	Sometimes	Often
I feel threatened here.	Never	Sometimes	Often
I wake up wishing that I were home.	Never	Sometimes	Often
I made a mistake moving here.	Never	Sometimes	Often
I feel lonely here.	Never	Sometimes	Often

VALIDATION

Test-retest Reliability

The measure of homesickness involves a state characteristic in that it is a specific response to a transition involving leaving home. Also adaptation to the new environment will occur and therefore the level of homesickness may well be expected to change with time. Therefore test-retest correlations would be expected to vary within and between subjects, and are inappropriate. Only the non-homesick would be expected to show a stable response pattern. A retest on 34 non-homesick and 54 homesick student subjects gave a retest correlation coefficient of 0.71 and 0.59 respectively across two weeks, and 0.81 and 0.21 respectively across six months. All correlation coefficients were significant statistically at at least $p < 0.05$. This implies that the state of non-homesickness is stable whereas the state of homesickness is not stable.

Construct Validation

In order to show that a questionnaire has construct validity it must be shown to measure what it claims to measure, namely, in this case, 'homesickness'. Unfortunately, unlike the situation for clinical disorders, there are no groups of individuals diagnosed by professionals available. Therefore there is no way to establish a criterion group in order to establish that they score high on the inventory.

A major problem lay in obtaining some other source of independent assessment. Students and pupils may not readily admit to homesickness and with the exception of extreme cases, the outward signs may be confined to private moments and are not easily revealed to observers.

Initial results of a school-based study have however provided some hopeful data. In a sample of 31 boarding school pupils aged 11–13, each pupil completed the DRI and was independently rated for signs of homesickness by a housemaster. The correlation coefficient was 0.40, ($p < 0.02$). Unfortunately, the same study could not be repeated using university staff.

SUMMARY AND CONCLUSIONS

This Appendix has provided the basic data on the design of a state measure for assessing homesickness following transition from home into residence at a school or university. Although four factors ('adaptation'; 'home'; 'satisfaction' and 'social') were identified from initial responses to generated questions, the items which predicted items were those concerned with cognitions centred on 'home'.

The questionnaire cannot easily be validated in the conventional way because of the lack of existing research data on homesickness and the lack of diagnosed criterion groups who could be asked to provide ratings. Some attempt has been made to provide data from those in custodial roles (schoolmasters, teachers, tutors, etc.) but there is no reason why a socially sanctioned experience thought by many to be a weakness should be indicated to authority figures. Some modest success was however obtained from data provided by boarding schoolmasters.

More data is now needed in order that the validity of the DRI can be further established. The author welcomes correspondence from any interested party who would like to help refine the validity of the inventory. One extra step which might prove helpful is to combine the DRI with the Middlesex Hospital Questionnaire scores (Crown & Crisp, 1966) in order that degree of distress can be taken into account.

References

Arredondo-Dowd, P. M. (1981). Personal loss and grief as a result of immigration. *The Personnel and Guidance Journal, 59*, 376–378.

Beck, A. T. (1967). *Depression: Clinical, experimental and theortical aspects*. New York: Harper & Row.

Beck, A. T. (1970). The core problem in depression. *Science and Psychoanalysis, 17*, 47–55.

Berkson, D. E. (1962). Mortality and marital status. Reflections on the derivation of etiology from statistics. *American Journal of Public Health, 52*, 1318.

Bills, A. (1931). Blocking: A new principle in mental fatigue. *American Journal of Psychology, 43*, 230–45.

Boman, B. (1988). Stress and heart disease. In S. Fisher & J. Reason (Eds.), *The handbook of life stress, cognition and health*. Chichester: John Wiley & Sons.

Bowlby, J. (1969). *Attachment and Loss. Vol. 1: Attachment*. New York: Basic Books.

Bowlby, J. (1973). *Attachment and Loss. Vol. 2: Separation, anxiety and anger*. New York: Basic Books.

Bowlby, J. (1980). *Attachment and Loss. Vol. 3: Loss, sadness and depression*. New York: Basic Books.

Broadbent, D. E. (1958). *Perception and communication*. London: Pergamon Press.

Broadbent, D. E., Cooper, P. F., Fitzgerald, P., & Parkes, K. R. (1982). The Cognitive Failures Questionnaire (CFQ) and its correlates. *British Journal of Clinical Psychology, 21*, 1–16.

Brown, G. (1974). Meaning, measurement and stress of life events. In B. S. Dohrenwend & B. P. Dohrenwend (Eds.), *Stressful life events: their nature and effects*. New York: Wiley.

Brown, G. W. (1988). Early loss of parent and depression in adult life. In S. Fisher & J. Reason, (Eds.), *The handbook of life stress, cognition and health*. Chichester: John Wiley & Sons.

Brown, G. W., & Harris, T. H. (1978). *The social origins of depression; A study of psychiatric disorders in women*. London: Tavistock.

Brown, I. (1964). The measurement of perceptual load and reserve capacity. *The Transactions of the Associations of Industrial Medical Officers, 14*, 44–49.

Brown, J., & Armstrong, M. (1986). Transfer from junior to secondary: The child's perspective. In M. B. Youngman (Ed.), *Mid-schooling transfer: Problems and proposals* (p.p. 29–46). Slough: NFER-Nelson.

Bugen, L. A. (1977). Human grief: a model for prediction and intervention. *American Journal of Orthopsychiatry 4*, 196–206.

Cameron, N. A., & Margaret, A. (1951). *Behaviour pathology*. New York: Houghton.

Christenson, W. W., & Hinkle, L. E. (1961). Differences in illnesses and prognostic signs in two groups of young men. *Journal of the American Medical Association, 177*, 247–253.

Claparede, E. (1934). *La genese de l'hypothese*. Geneva: Kundig.

Clochrane, R. (1983). *The social creation of mental illness*. New York: Longman (Applied Psychology Series).

Connolly, J. (1975). Circumstances events and illness. *Medicine, 2(10)*, 454–458.

Corp, R. (1791). An essay on the changes produced in the body by the operation of the mind, by the late Dr. Corp of Bath. (Reproduced in Ratner, D. J. (1958). *Mind and body in 18th century medicine*. London: Wellcome Historical Library.)

Crombag, H. F. M. (1968). *Studie motivatie en studie attitude*. Croningen: Walters.

Crown, S., & Crisp, A. H. (1966). A short clinical diagnostic self-rating for psycho-neurotic patients. *British Journal of Psychiatry, 112*, 917–923.

Cruze-Coke, R., Etcheverry, R., & Nagel, R. (1964). Influences of migration on blood pressure of Easter Islanders. *Lancet, March 28*, 697–699.

de Paulo, B. M., Brown, P. L., Ishie, S., & Fisher, J. D. (1981). Help that works: The effects of aid on subsequent task performance. *Personality and Social Psychology, 41*, 478–487.

Dodge, D. L., & Martin W. T. (1970). *Social stress and chronic illness: mortality patterns in industrial society*. London: University of Notre Dame Press.

Eysenck, M. (1988). Trait anxiety and stress. In S. Fisher & J. Reason, (Eds.), *The handbook of life stress, cognition and health*. Chichester: John Wiley & Sons.

Faris, R. E. L., & Dunham, H. W. (1939). *Mental disorders in urban areas: An ecological study of schizophrenia and other psychoses*. Chicago: Chicago University Press.

Fischer, C. S., & Stueve, C. A. (1977). 'Authentic community?': The role of place in modern life. In C. S. Fischer, R. M. Jackson, & C. A. Stueve et al. (Eds.), *Networks and places: Social relations in the urban setting*, (p.p. 163–186). New York: The Free Press.

Fisher, S. (1984). *Stress and the perception of control*. London: Lawrence Erlbaum Associates Ltd.

Fisher, S. (1985). Control and blue collar work. In C. L. Cooper & M. J. Smith (Eds.), *Job stress and blue collar work*. Chichester: John Wiley & Sons.

Fisher, S. (1986). *Stress and Strategy*. London: Lawrence Erlbaum Associates Ltd.

Fisher, S. (1987). Methodological factors in the investigation of stress and health at work. In J. Hurrell, S. Salter & C. Cooper (Eds.), *Methodological factors in occupational stress*. London: Taylor & Francis Ltd.

Fisher, S. (1988a). Life stress, control strategies and the risk of disease: A psychobiological model. In S. Fisher & J. Reason (Eds.), *Handbook of life stress, cognition and health*. Chichester: John Wiley & Sons.

Fisher, S. (1988b). Stress, control and the implications for health at work. In S. Salter, J. Hurrell, & C. Cooper (Eds.), *Job control and worker health*. Chichester: John Wiley & Sons. (In press).

Fisher, S., Frazer, N., & Murray, K. (1984). The transition from home to boarding school: a diary-style analysis of the problems and worries of boarding school pupils. *Journal of Environmental Psychology, 4*, 211–221.

Fisher, S., Frazer, N., & Murray, K. (1986). Homesickness and health in boarding school children. *Journal of Environmental Psychology, 6*, 35–37

Fisher, S., & Frazer, N. The stress of transition to nursing college. *British Journal of Psychology*, (submitted for publication).

Fisher, S., & Hood, B. (1987). The stress of the transition to university: a longitudinal study of vulnerability to psychological disturbance and homesickness. *British Journal of Psychology, 78*, 425–441.

Fisher, S., & Hood, B. (1988). Vulnerability factors in the transition to university: self-reported mobility history and sex differences as factors in psychological disturbance. *British Journal of Psychology, 79*, 1–13.

Fisher, S., Murray, K., & Frazer, N. (1985). Homesickness and health in first-year students. *Journal of Environmental Psychology, 5*, 181–195.

Fisher, S., Elder, L., & Peacock, G. Circumstantial determinants of homesickness incidence. *Work and Stress*, (submitted for publication).

Fisher, S., & Reason, J. (1988). *The handbook of life stress cognition and health*. Chichester: John Wiley & Sons.

Frankenhaeuser, M., & Johansson, J. (1982). Stress at work: Psychobiological and psychosocial aspects. *Paper presented at the 20th International Conference of Applied Psychology*. Edinburgh: July 25–31.

French, J. R. P., Caplan, R., & Van Harrison, R. (Eds.) (1982). *The mechanics of job stress and strain*. New York: John Wiley & Sons.

Fried, M. (1962). Grieving for a lost home, In L. J. Duhl (Ed.), *The Environment of the Metropolis*. New York: Basic Books.

Gilbert, P. (1988). The psychobiology of depression. In S. Fisher & J. Reason (Eds.), *The handbook of life stress, cognition and health*. Chichester & New York: John Wiley & Sons.

Greenwald, A. G. (1970). Sensory feedback mechanisms in performance control: With special reference to the ideomotor mechanism. *Psychological Review, 77*, 73–99.

Hamilton, V. (1974). Socialisation anxiety and information processing: A capacity model of anxiety-induced performance deficits. *Paper presented at a conference on the Dimensions of Anxiety and Stress*. Athens, Greece: September.

Harder, J. J. (1678). *Dissertio medico de nostalgia order heinweh praeside*. Basle: Johannes Heferno.

Hojat M., & Herman, M. W. (1985). Adjustment and psychosocial problems of Iranian and Filipino physicians in the U.S. *Journal of Clinical Psychology, 41*, 130–136.

Holmes, T. H., & Rahe, R. H. (1965). The social readjustment rating scale. *Journal of Psychosomatic Research, 11*, 213–218.

Hood, B., MacLachlan, M., & Fisher, S. (1987). The relationship between cognitive failures, psychoneurotic symptoms and sex. *Acta Psychiatrica Scandinavia, 76*, 33–35.

Hormuth, S. (1984). Transitions in commitments to roles and self-concept change: Relocation as a paradigm. In V. L. Allen & E. Van de Vlert (Eds.), *Role transitions: Explorations and explanations*. New York: Plenum.

Howarth, I., & Dootjes Dussuyer, I. (1988). Helping people cope with the long-term effects of stress. In S. Fisher & J. Reason (Eds.), *Handbook of life stress, cognition and health*. Chichester: John Wiley & Sons.

Jastrow, J. (1905). The lapses of consciousness. *The Popular Science Monthly, LXVII–31*, 481–502.

Kane, G. (1987). *Studies of coping in stressed populations*. Dissertation for the degree of Doctor of Philosophy at the University of Manchester, U.K.

Karasek, R. A. (1979). Job demands, job decision latitude and mental strain; implication for job redesign. *Administrative Science Quarterly, 24*, 285–309.

Kleiner, R. J., & Parker, S. (1963). Goal-striving and psychosomatic symptoms in a migrant and non-migrant population. In M. B. Kantor (Ed.), *Mobility and Mental Health*. Springfield, Illinois: Charles C. Thomson.

Klinger, E. (1975). Consequences of commitment to and disengagement from incentives. *Psychological Review, 82,(1)*, 1–7.

Kuhl, J., & Kazen-Saad, M. (1988). A motivational approach to volition: Activation and de-activation of memory representations related to uncompleted intentions. In V. Hamilton, G. H. Bower, & N. Frijda (Eds.), *Cognition, emotion and affect: A cognitive science view.* Dordrecht: Martinas Nijhoff Publishing.

Lazarus, R. S., & Folkman, S. (1984). *Stress, appraisal and coping.* New York: Springer.

Leff, M. J., Roatch, J. F., & Bunney, W. E. (1970). Environmental factors preceding the onset of severe depressions. *British Journal of Psychiatry, 33*, 293–311.

Lindemann, E. (1944). The symptomatology and management of acute grief. *American Journal of Psychiatry, 101*, 141–148.

Lloyd, G. G., & Lishman, W. A. (1975). Effects of depression on the speed of recall of pleasant and unpleasant experiences. *Psychological Medicine, 5*, 173–180.

Loeb, A., Beck, A., & Diggory, J. (1971). Differential effects of success and failure on depressed and non-depressed patients. *The Journal of Nervous and Mental Disease, 152, 2*, 106–113.

Malzberg, B., & Lee, E. S. (1940). *Migration and mental disease: A study of first admissions to hospital for mental disease.* New York: Social Science Research Council.

Mandler, G. (1975). *Mind and emotion.* New York: John Wiley & Sons.

Mandler, G., & Watson, D. L. (1966). Anxiety and the interruption of behaviour. In C. D. Spielberger (Ed.) *Anxiety and behaviour*, New York: Academic Press.

Medalie, J. H., & Kahn, H. A. (1973). Myocardial infraction over a five-year period. I: Prevalence, incidence and mortality experience. *Journal of Chronic Diseases, 26*, 63–84.

Michelson, W. (1976). *Man and his urban environment: A socio-biological approach* (2nd Ed.). Reading, Mass.: Addison-Wesley.

Miller, J. G. (1962). Adjusting to overloads of information. In D. Rioch & E. Weinstein (Eds.), *Disorders of communication.* New York: Hafner Publishing Company.

Miller, G., Galanter, E., & Pribram, K. (1960). *Plans and the structure of behavior.* New York: Holt Rinehart & Winston.

Mowrer, O. H., & Viek, P. (1948). An experimental analogue of fear from a sense of helplessness. *Journal of Abnormal Social Psychology, 43*, 193–200.

Nicassio, P. M., & Pate, J. K. (1984). An analysis of problems of resettlement of the Indochinese refugees in the U.S. *Social Psychiatry, 19*, 135–141.

Oatley, K. (1988). Life events, social cognition and depression. In S. Fisher & J. Reason (Eds.), *Handbook of life stress, cognition and health.* Chichester: John Wiley & Sons.

Oatley, K., & Bolton. W. (1985). A social cognitive theory of depression in relation to life events. *Psychological Review, 92, 3*, 372–388.

Odegaard, O. (1932). Emigration and insanity: A study of mental disease among the Norwegian born population of Minnesota. *Acta Psychiatrica et Neurologica*, Supplement, 1–4.

Parkes, C. M. (1965). Bereavement and mental illness. *British Journal of Medical Psychology, 38*, 1–26.

Parkes, C. M. (1972). *Bereavement.* New York: International University Press.

Peacock, G. (1988). *Homesickness.* PhD thesis, La Trobe University, Melbourne, Australia.

Rahe, R. (1988). Recent life changes and coronary heart disease. In S. Fisher & J. Reason (Eds.), *The handbook of life stress, cognition and health.* Chichester: John Wiley & Sons.

Rapaport, D. (1961). Emotions and memory. *The Menninger Clinic Monograph Series. No. 2.* New York: Science Editions.

Reason, J. (1976). Absent minds. *New Society*, 4, 244–245.

Reason, J. (1977). Skill and error in everyday life. In M. Howe (Ed.), *Adult Learning.* London: John Wiley & Sons.

Reason, J. T., & Lucas, D. (1982). *The short inventory of mental lapses (SIML).* Unpublished report: University of Manchester.

Ryle, A. (1982). Psychotherapy: A cognitive integration of theory and practice. London: Academic Press.

Schönpflug, W., & Batman, W. (1988). The costs and benefits of coping. In S. Fisher & J. Reason (Eds.), *The handbook of life stress, cognition & health.* Chichester: John Wiley & Sons.

Selye, H. (1974). *Stress without distress.* Philadelphia and New York: Lippincott.

Stokols, D. (1979). A congruence analysis of human stress. In I. G. Sarason & C. D. Spielberger (Eds.), *Stress and anxiety, Vol. 6.* New York: John Wiley & Sons.

Stokols, D., Schumaker, S. A., & Martinez, J. (1983). Residential mobility and pesonal well-being. *Journal of Environmental Psychology, 3,* 5–19.

Syme, S. L. (1967). Implications and future prospects. In S. L. Syme and L. G. Reeder (Eds.), *Social stress and cardio vascular disease.* Milbank Memorial Fund Quarterly.

Tausk V. (1969). On the psychology of the war deserter. *The Psychoanalytic Quarterly,* Volume 38, no. 3, 354–381.

Torbjorn, I. (1982). *Living abroad.* New York: John Wiley & Sons.

Totman, R. (1979). *Social Causes of Illness.* London: Souvenir Press.

Van Harrison, R. (1978). Person-environment fit and job stress. In C. L. Cooper & R. Payne (Eds.), *Stress at work.* London: John Wiley & Sons.

Von Holst, E. (1954). Relation between the central nervous system and the peripheral organs. *British Journal of Animal Behaviour, 2,* 89–94.

Wapner, S., Kaplan, B., & Ciottone, R. (1981). Self-world relationships in critical environmental transitions: Childhood and beyond. In L. S. Liben, A. H. Patterson, & N. Newcombe (Eds.), *Spatial representations and behaviour across the life span.* New York: Academic Press.

Weiss, J. M. (1968). Effects of coping responses on stress. *Journal of Comparative and Physiological Psychology, 65,* 251–266.

Weiss, J. M. (1970). Somatic effects of predictable and unpredictable shock. *Psychosomatic Medicine, 32,* 397–408.

Weiss, R. (1975). *Marital separation.* New York: Basic Books.

Weiss, R. (1978). Couples' relationships. In M. Corbin (Ed.), *The couple.* New York: Penguin.

Weiss, R. (1982). Attachment in adult life. In C. M. Parkes & J. Stevenson-Hinde (Eds.), *The place of attachment and loss in human behaviour.* London: Tavistock Press.

Wherry, R. J., & Curran, P. M. (1965). A study of some determinants of psychological stress. *U.S. Naval School of Aviation Medicine Report,* July.

Wickland, R. A. (1975). Objective self-awareness. In L. Berkowitz (Ed.), *Advances in experimental social psychology,* Vol. 8, (233–275). New York: Academic Press.

Wolff, H. G. (1953). *Stress and disease.* Springfield, Illinois: Charles C. Thomas.

Zuckert, J. F. (1768). *Von den Liedenschafen.* Berlin. (Cited in Rather, 1958.)

Author Index

Subject Index

Absent-mindedness, 50–56
Addiction, 92
Anxiety, xiii, 37–39, 30–34, 60–65
Attention, 42–48, 75–78, 111–122

Bereavement, xiii, 10–14, 22, 24, 118–119

Circumstantial effects of moves, 3–6, 67–69, 72–74
Cognitive failure, (*see* absent-mindedness)
Commitment, 96–99, 111–112, 120–121
Competing demands model, 42–48, 75–78, 111–112
Conflict, 18–19, 61
Congruence, 6–7, 14, 110–111
Control theory, xiv, 12–18, 22, 58–63
Culture shock, 2–6; 73–74

Demand, 60, 75–78, 100–103
Depression, 10–108, 22, 24, 58–65, 89–92, 120–121, 123–141
Disease, 59–60
Distress (*see also* Homesickness), 37–39, 30–34, 60–65, 123–141

Dundee relocation inventory, 49, 123–141

Epidemiological problem analysis, 103

Grief, xiii, 10–14, 22, 24, 118–119

Health, 2–8, 11–12, 22, 49–54, 57–65
Homesickness
    Background factors in, 74
    Biological models of, 107–109
    Cognitive factors in, xii, 39–48, 81–94, 96–104, 107–117
    Composite models of, 107–117
    Definitions of, 21–22, 30–34,
    Early texts on, 23–24
    Incidence of, xiii, 25–30, 34, 37–39
    Measurement of, 123–141
    Personal aspects of, xii, 30–36, 69–72
    Phenomenology of, 21–35
    Satisfaction, 69–70, 78–79,
    Social desirability and, 26–27

Ideomotor theory, 13–14

151